Integrating Yoga and Play Therapy

of related interest

Fun Games and Physical Activities to Help Heal Children Who Hurt
Get On Your Feet!
Beth Powell, LCSW
ISBN 978 1 78592 773 7
eISBN 978 1 78450 678 0

Integrating Art Therapy and Yoga Therapy
Yoga, Art, and the Use of Intention
Karen Gibbons
ISBN 978 1 84905 782 0
eISBN 978 1 78450 023 8

Play and Art in Child Psychotherapy
An Expressive Arts Therapy Approach
Ellen G. Levine
ISBN 978 1 84905 504 8
eISBN 978 0 85700 919 7

Mindful Little Yogis
Self-Regulation Tools to Empower Kids with Special Needs to Breathe and Relax
Nicola Harvey
Illustrated by John Smisson
ISBN 978 1 84819 404 5
eISBN 978 0 85701 360 6

Teen Yoga for Yoga Therapists
A Guide to Development, Mental Health and Working with Common Teen Issues
Charlotta Martinus
Foreword by Sir Anthony Seldon
ISBN 978 1 84819 399 4
eISBN 978 0 85701 355 2

Integrating Yoga and Play Therapy

THE MIND–BODY APPROACH FOR HEALING ADVERSE CHILDHOOD EXPERIENCES

MICHELLE PLISKE AND LINDSAY BALBOA

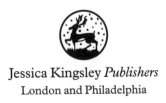

Jessica Kingsley *Publishers*
London and Philadelphia

First published in 2019
by Jessica Kingsley Publishers
73 Collier Street
London N1 9BE, UK
and
400 Market Street, Suite 400
Philadelphia, PA 19106, USA

www.jkp.com

Library of Congress Cataloging in Publication Data
Names: Pliske, Michelle, author. | Balboa, Lindsay, author.
Title: Integrating yoga and play therapy : the mind body approach for healing
  adverse childhood experiences / Michelle Pliske and Lindsay Balboa.
Description: London ; Philadelphia : Jessica Kingsley Publishers, 2019. |
  Includes bibliographical references and index.
Identifiers: LCCN 2018050531 | ISBN 9781785928123
Subjects: | MESH: Child Behavior Disorders--therapy | Yoga--psychology | Play
  Therapy | Psychological Trauma--therapy | Child | Case Reports
Classification: LCC RJ505.P6 | NLM WS 350.7 | DDC 618.92/891653-
-dc23 LC record available at https://lccn.loc.gov/2018050531

British Library Cataloguing in Publication Data
A CIP catalogue record for this book is available from the British Library

ISBN 978 1 78592 812 3
eISBN 978 1 78450 868 5

Printed and bound in the United States

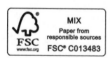

Dedication

To my spouse Gregory with love. Your unconditional love, support and care has made this work and life possible.

—*Michelle Pliske*

To the children and families who have welcomed me and allowed me to be their helper. I am honored to have grown alongside you throughout the years.

—*Lindsay Balboa*

Contents

Acknowledgments 9

Disclaimer 11

Introduction. 13

1. A Primer on Child Development, Play and
   Expressive Arts Therapies 23

2. The Mind–Body Connection: Yoga and Play to Address
   Adverse Experiences for Children 47

3. Non-Directive and Directive Yoga and Play Therapy Practice:
   Case Examples: Kelly, Anna and Emily 97

4. Yoga and Play Can Happen in Every Setting:
   Group and Family Systems 135

5. Concluding Thoughts: Self-Care and Future Research 157

References 169

Further Reading 181

About the Authors 183

Subject Index 185

Author Index 189

Acknowledgments

There are many people who have helped shape me throughout my career. First, my family who has supported me every step of the way. My spouse, Gregory, mother-in-law, Margaret, and children, Lily, David and Dahlia, who have supported me through providing words of encouragement and love daily. I want to thank my parents, who have encouraged me all throughout my education and life's adventures and kindly remind me to take care of myself every time we talk. I would also like to acknowledge all my colleagues at Firefly. The laughter and words of encouragement, as well as critical peer feedback, not only challenges me to grow but has been, and continues to be, a foundational support for moving forward in this field. Their wisdom, expertise and thoughtful reflections impact my work greatly in such a positive way. No clinician stands alone, we stand on the shoulders of giants. I acknowledge all the great work in this collaborative field of neuroscientists, child developmental psychologists, play therapists, social workers and counselors. We disseminate research and education so that others can learn and contribute new ideas to the field. I want to acknowledge Imagination Yoga for their amazing contribution of innovative ways to engage children in yoga. I thank and extend appreciation and many thanks to my mentors throughout my career: Susan Hedlund, Dawn Williamson, Jessica Ritter and Sara Webb. All are brilliant clinicians and researchers who inspired me to work harder, think more critically and deeply, all while living life wholeheartedly. Lastly, I want to extend my sincere gratitude and thanks to Lindsay Balboa, the co-author of this text. She consistently demonstrates excellence in the field with her dedication to preventing child abuse and supporting those impacted by trauma and adversity. She simply brings a bright light of hope into this world.

—Michelle Pliske

There are many folks I would also like to thank for supporting me throughout my adventure through life and my career thus far. Mom and Dad, thanks for not completely freaking out when I decided I wanted to be a social worker instead of a doctor. Dad, thanks for letting me bring home all the stray animals and allowing me to give them a loving home, while also continuously reminding me of the importance of showing the same love to myself. Thanks to Thomas for your logic, love and humor. Thanks to my army of in-laws for welcoming me with open arms and taking me in as one of your own. I couldn't ask for a better group of humans in my life.

Sydney and Cecilia, you are both my little lights.

Thanks to my friends for being amazingly talented and reminding me of our endless power and ability to accomplish all tasks in front of us.

Thank you to my colleagues, current and past, who have taught me and held space for me when our work has been heavy.

Last, but not least, I would like to thank Michelle for taking me under her wing and seeing something in me that caused her to think I would be a great co-author and partner in crime. You believe in me and constantly encourage me to be better than I was yesterday, and I am forever appreciative. I would not be the professional I am today without you and Greg, and I look forward to our future adventures.

—Lindsay Balboa

Disclaimer

Standards of clinical practice evolve over time; therefore, no technique or recommendation is guaranteed to be safe or effective in all circumstances. This work is intended to provide general information as a resource for professionals practicing within the field of mental health; it is not a substitute for comprehensive training on neurobiology, body systems including movement, yoga, or play therapy. We recommend coursework, training and appropriate peer mentorship and supervision when engaging in clinical practice that involves child psychotherapy, expressive arts and movement-based interventions which comply with the clinician's code of ethics. Neither the publisher nor the authors can guarantee the complete accuracy, efficacy or appropriateness of any recommendation provided within this text for every circumstance. Aspects of case history have been altered or changed for confidentiality and privacy.

Introduction

Much of the credit for integrating movement and play therapy goes directly to our clients. We feel privileged to walk alongside our kids as they navigate some of the most complex issues facing humanity. Human suffering can bring pain and sorrow; however, children somehow manage to find the ability to see love, create new beginnings and inherently know what is needed if we only stop to listen. Eliana Gil once presented at a national conference in which she stated "let children lead the way," which resonated with us. Children do lead the way and show us that what is needed cannot be constricted; they need to have the opportunity to physically move within the therapeutic process, guiding their own narrative throughout, with the use of physical movement, art and play. The importance of therapists cannot be overstated as they are responsible for creating a holding environment, or the relationship's emotional safety and trust, a construct developed by English pediatrician and psychoanalyst Donald Winnicott. This holding environment creates a safe physical and psychological space to allow freedom of expression, spontaneous interactions and opportunity for self-exploration (Flanagan 2016a). We emphasize the therapist as being integral to the outcome of trauma treatment. Therapists are vital to the change process; they have the power and importance to create a secure base for children, facilitate exploration and serve as a co-regulator during times of reprocessing trauma, thereby helping build the necessary regulation skills to become autocatalytic for the child in the future.

Our goal is to create the best possible environment for meeting the needs of clients and therapists alike. This is a fundamental principle founding the institute where the authors of this text practice. We continue to develop policies and practice standards for clients seeking care and clinicians seeking professional development. A teenage client long ago suggested the name Firefly while I (Michelle) was working within a hospice setting. Toward the end of our grief and bereavement work, the client brought in a canvas of a night sky, painted at home, which held one pinprick of brilliant light in the center. She said that losing her mother to stage-four breast cancer was a time of utter darkness in which she had felt hopeless and helpless to move forward. She created a canvas titled "The Firefly in the Night" to represent her time in therapy as a single point of hope, symbolizing her grief and loss work. We believe that as a community of therapists we can provide a space of healing to those we serve, and that space should concurrently support the therapist as well. As we formulated how to build an institute for children and families it was important to have the space built and centered on these principles, ensuring we can continue to have room for children to thrive. This included creating large, open offices allowing for unrestricted movement and filled with opportunities to engage in creativity and play through having ample choices in the play and art materials provided. Play occurs in conjunction with a therapist's willingness to be present and vulnerable. We built a space where therapists can feel challenged professionally to continue learning; mastering theory and clinical applications as well as receiving necessary peer feedback and ongoing support.

Connection

We argue that trauma work with children must include the components of the body for creating a mind–body connection to integrate adverse experiences to find new meanings associated with the past and shift perspective in a manner which allows healing from a holistic approach. This requires connection within the playroom. Brown (2010) defines connection as the energy which exists among people when they feel seen, heard and valued; when someone can give and receive without judgment and can obtain strength from the relationship. The way in which we connect with children requires us to be vulnerable, and we must enter the playroom knowing our own experiences and histories. Inherently our past and present collide, the way we manage our emotions and systems in conjunction with the child for co-regulation supports attunement, and this becomes the catalyst for connection to occur between the child and therapist.

Adversity and society

Exposure to early childhood adversity including abuse and trauma is not a new phenomenon, nor is it a phenomenon unique to developing worlds. Children have been exposed to numerous forms of maltreatment throughout human history, including being viewed as possessions and/or a source of labor or income, with socioeconomic status often determining the life course of a child (Costin 1997; Gil 1991; Johnson 2015). Throughout history, children have been exposed to death, famine and war within their communities or even been witness to public punishments or executions.

Child mental health professionals understand that childhood exposure to violence is not new and is experienced globally; however, recovery has been tied to the strength of relationship, community and ritual. The significance of ritual and community is demonstrated in the research of children who return home after experiences with war in northern Uganda. A key aspect discussed in this research includes community variables which mitigate trauma symptoms, such as the tribal community's ability for reintegration of children back into their village with understanding, care and support (Pham, Vinck and Stover 2009). A reunion met with shame or disgust, lacking support, results in children experiencing higher overall trauma symptoms and difficult recoveries. It can be considered a universal phenomenon that children who experience violence, abuse, war and suffering coupled with isolation and shame will undoubtedly struggle as a result.

The last few decades have brought a shift in the way we experience childhood. The delivery of trauma exposure for children has evolved with added violence embedded within everyday media.

Graphic representations of human suffering have become common occurrences within news, film, music, social media and other internet platforms, thereby creating a society which experiences fear and uncertainty. Presently, we hear parents expressing this fear citing concerns about allowing their children to have free movement within neighborhoods and communities. This results in more children becoming confined to homes or apartments in isolation. Children isolated at home, coupled with advances in technology, allow engagement with media as a means of entertainment. Overuse of this media in pediatric populations carries consequences such as exposure to violence, loneliness, low self-esteem, low social competence and low life satisfaction. This is due to a lack of real-world interactions and reduced opportunities for creativity and exercise or physical movement (Lemmens, Valkenburg and Peter 2011).

Educators in the United States have been driven towards creating higher performance outcomes on standardized testing for children. The outcome is the sacrifice of educational creativity, and the loss of our educator's independence in finding ways of meeting children's learning needs within the classroom. The push towards standardized testing shifts funding away from the arts and creativity within education practice to support testing success. Teachers are also forced into larger and larger classroom sizes which limit their time and energy. Children spend a vast amount of their development in the classroom. Teachers are doing the best they can, but are often unable to find time for developing unique ways of connecting with kids who may need a higher level of intervention and management due to their individually unique experiences with adversity and trauma. Exposure to violence, fear, neglect and adversity can disrupt learning and the ability to physically regulate emotion. What we see is stress within society increasing, while resources within classrooms and homes are decreasing.

A parallel argument with the education system can be made to the field of children's mental health. Managed care has also created complexity for therapists who provide mental health support. Insurance companies are driving the way we deliver care by pushing manualized evidence-based treatment methods for reimbursement related to diagnosis. There are insurance programs which front-load sums of money to providers based on the diagnosis upon assessment. Providers become rewarded if they use a short-term, manualized treatment model, thereby discharging the client more quickly and increasing their monetary outcome. Providers who need to continue working with clients beyond the front-loaded sum, find themselves penalized, audited and questioned for not producing results more quickly. Systems like this can breed corruption and need scrutiny from legislators and policy makers. Manualized models can stifle therapeutic creativity and lack opportunity for the provider to be flexible and develop individually unique plans to meet the needs of a child. This cookbook therapy model is anathema to the reality of solutions found in creative arts and play therapy. Expressive arts and life in general are complex and varied: one size does not fit all.

Managed care has created scenarios in which it can feel necessary to build provider calendars with back-to-back scheduled clients to make ends meet, due to financial reductions in session reimbursement. Therapists can feel the stress and pressure of an "evidence-based world" and we can be expected by employers or managed care companies to complete treatment in a brief model. This type of program within managed care was not the intention when evidence-based practice was adopted for achieving mental health competencies for providers' outcomes in client care. Evidence-based practice includes practice-based wisdom. Organized psychiatry has transformed the way we think over the last few decades, yet we see mainstream news reports and academic journals detailing the corrupting influence of pharmaceutical money within modern medicine and mental health service delivery (Whitaker and Cosgrove 2015). We have listened to account after account of therapists expressing both concern and frustration with managed care, pharmaceutical influence and fear around treatment plans being denied as they are not evidence-based "enough". There lies the pressure to move quickly in therapy, because the consequence may be a loss of financial support from insurance institutions. Our hope is to help shift thinking away from limited or rigid designs centered on fear toward a conversation which includes understanding that there are evidence and practice-informed models of care to address pediatric mental health issues which transcend manualized treatment formats.

Holding space for children who suffer

Child therapists are often asked to intervene to support family systems and communities in crisis. The toll for this work can often be felt somatically for therapists, as therapists manage stress and bear witness to human suffering. This can also sometimes occur while living within the very communities which are impacted by poverty, violence or disaster. We stated how connection is a key component of trauma work; therefore service to those who suffer inevitably involves absorbing pain associated with the suffering, creating a condition known as secondary traumatic stress (Newell and MacNeil 2010). We ask the question: How do we engage in this work while simultaneously supporting the prospect for long-term work in the field? Combining movement and creative expression within sessions is a vital component to addressing this question. This combination occurs in conjunction with therapists monitoring their own physiological state to co-regulate the child, and having opportunities to process session content within a professional community. Not practicing alone offers the ability to manage and mitigate secondary traumatic stress through relationship with peers and consultation. We argue therapists are the most important aspect of implementing therapy and it is difficult to be a child trauma therapist working alone; this work is best done in a community, ensuring the therapist has ongoing support so that they, in turn, can support their clients.

The authors of this text have tailored their education and centered their careers around understanding child development. This includes infant toddler mental health, attachment theory, learning theories, developmental theories, neurobiology and how childhood developmental adversity or trauma impacts every aspect of a child. Monumental to our learning has been Bruce Perry's work with the neurosequential model of therapeutics (NMT) (Perry 2006). Expressive arts in therapy are defined as "action therapies" (Weiner 1999), such as art, drama and movement through dance or yoga, which help individuals explore issues and communicate thoughts and feelings. All forms of drama, creative writing, music-making and play include participatory and sensory experiences in which individuals invest energy (Malchiodi 2008). Art, drama and movement provide nonverbal strategies for communicating thoughts, feelings or experiences. The documentary *Paper Tigers* (KPJR Films Production 2015) profiles a high school and group of teenagers who have been exposed to significant adversity and trauma. This documentary depicts not only relational factors which contribute to positive outcomes in youth facing adversity, but relationships embedded within expressive arts, including music, movement, drama, art and wilderness-based experiences. The connection of expressive arts within this documentary is often missed, where it is drawing upon the ability to process complex trauma in a way that derives meaning through relationship. This integration of creative expression coupled with relationship provides opportunities for resiliency to form.

What stands out for us in reflection of the culmination of theory, science and clinical practice is the importance of connection within relationship. We argue that working with adversity and trauma cannot be done without having a relationship with your client. This includes attunement and the ability to be vulnerable, meaning we need to be able to have comfort within our own body. We need to know our own experiences to help another person allow their body to integrate and process complex adversity and trauma. Relationship includes the therapist doing their own work to gain understanding of past experiences and how this comes into the room within a session. Relationship includes the therapist having a community of support to help protect against toxic exposure to stress and vicarious trauma by having the ability to diffuse the emotion within a group who are ready to help detoxify it (Bloom 2013). Relationship with a traumatized child requires multi-faceted layers of intervention and support provided by a highly educated therapist working within a community.

Holding space for children who suffer include offerings of creative interventions through movement which encourage externalization. We achieve this by exploring a trauma narrative and the associated feelings derived from an adverse experience through combining art and movement (Malchiodi 2008). The key to supporting a traumatized child is creating safety and utilizing somatosensory routes within the process. This can include repetitive rhythmic movement, music or allowing art and creative expression to unfold through play (Gaskill and Perry 2014). Traditional methods, which include highly cognitive or heavy language-based approaches (top-down approaches), are likely to fail with children exposed to complex trauma when the lower brain networks are disorganized, underdeveloped or impaired; therefore providing bottom-up approaches (music, movement, drawing, play) allows children the ability to make meaning of adversity and counter-condition the effects of toxic stress (Gaskill and Perry 2014). The reality of therapy is that it is incredibly complex, as the human experience is complex. There is no one-size-fits-all approach to treatment and every child is different within their therapeutic process. Trauma therapists need time for thorough extended assessments and enough training and clinical supervision to successfully make sense of the case complexities. Therapists need support from managed care and their community for the time it takes unpack the layers of a child's experience, and training and education in neurobiology, supporting counseling theory applications into practice. Specialized training in expressive arts, along with ongoing consultation and peer support, is necessary to manage the vicarious effects of trauma and stress created by holding space for another's suffering. Successful outcomes include an intricate approach of incorporating all these components with consideration for cultural, racial and ethnic diversity. These aspects are critical for the child's integrated experience and acquired skills to autocatalytically become a self-sustaining regulation experience. Developing an autocatalytic outcome for a child provides opportunity to move forward in their life without the therapist's ongoing input, thus being able to find mastery in life.

Intentions for this text

We came to develop the paradigm of integrating movement and play as described in this text through our direct clinical work, client contributions, research of neurobiologically informed practices, knowledge of therapeutic play, art and our understanding of the importance of creating connections within relationship. The text will begin by building a platform for the conjunction of movement through yoga and play.

Chapter 1 will provide a brief primer for child development and include the historical knowledge of play therapy and art. This chapter is designed to draw a connection between play and art, keeping in mind the past knowledge and history of our field. We will discuss using play and art as a vehicle to put theory into practice, supported by research demonstrating the positive impact that play therapy brings to children's mental health issues.

Chapter 2 is designed to move us into a description of adverse childhood experiences and provides a rationale for the mind–body connection created by movement and expressive therapies. Trauma is defined utilizing current neuroscience and research which provides an answer for why trauma has such a physical and enduring behavioral effect. This chapter will introduce yoga and play therapy for a trauma-informed service delivery methodology.

Chapter 3 engages the reader in how to incorporate yoga and play therapy within non-directive and directive clinical practice sessions. This chapter will provide directive and non-directive approaches for bringing yoga into play therapy practice. Additionally, we will highlight how clinicians can help children create yoga narratives creating clarity for perceived challenges.

Chapter 4 focuses on how to create a highly structured plan for the specialized nature of group work or engaging in yoga and play or in larger family systems. This work can happen in a variety of settings and will include consideration for the dynamic nature of systems.

Chapter 5 concludes the text with discussion about continued areas of growth for specialization in the field and next steps for continued study to further professional growth. The chapter ends by acknowledging that the therapist, as an integral part of the treatment process, will require self-care in order to sustain clinical work over time.

Much of our work in this text is an integration and adaptation of theory and clinical applications. We seek to bring our professional histories, client experiences and current understanding of science into fruition by creating a model for supporting children who have experienced adversity and trauma. This text can by no means describe every aspect of child development or the neurobiology of trauma. Its aim does not include an in-depth understanding of play therapy or the philosophy underlying yoga practice. We seek to expand on foundational principles of play therapy and yoga and integrate modern sciences in a way that provides the ability for a therapist to utilize movement and play safely within the clinical setting. We want to emphasize that this text alone should not replace the education, training and supervision required to engage children in play therapy or yoga; however, we hope it inspires those to continue their own professional growth and development as this approach can profoundly change the lives of children who are impacted by trauma.

CHAPTER 1

A Primer on Child Development, Play and Expressive Arts Therapies

Child development

The history of childhood has gaps within its documentation and as a subject it historically has not been given enough attention. This may result from the actuality that children and women's lives have not been as well recorded as men's (Meadows 2018). The field of child development and psychology asserts that what we know about children is based on the historical knowledge and research of what is being prescribed as appropriate for child-rearing. It asserts interventions for pediatric populations; however, these continue to have a wide range of perspectives dependent upon culture, customs or norms (Stearns 2015).

Throughout this chapter we'll be discussing historical child development models and intervention styles. Specific considerations for therapeutic approach to intervention with child and parent support must take into consideration all aspects of current society, culture and memberships to various minority or majority communities. Anthropologists and behavioral scientists discuss culture including the full range of learned human behaviors, patterns or schemas. Practicing with cultural humility is necessary as we reflect upon intervention choices which draw upon historical contexts of theory and research. Cultural humility is a stance requiring a commitment to lifelong learning, continuous self-reflection and challenging one's own assumptions, beliefs, practices or comfort with not knowing or the unknown (Tervalon and Murray-Garcia 1998). We must recognize the power or privilege which exists in the room whether we are working with parents, children or family systems, a power that exists between clients and health professionals. Our goal is to approach another with openness, kindness and the willingness to learn—striving to understand rather than a stance of informing others what we think or know.

Children's behavior, expression of emotion and experience are shaped from the time of conception and during prenatal development through birth by the family's cultural norms, values and practice. Adults may unconsciously or consciously hold sets of beliefs or patterns (schemas) which carry enormous power for long-term development of the nervous system and cognitive processes (Taylor and Workman 2018). We will unpack the leading historical developmental models and theories for typical child development, knowing that child development lives within the context of the individual within the environment and is influenced by complex biological, social and cultural norms and expectations.

Child developmental periods can be divided into phases or ages capturing dramatic change and growth. It is not uncommon for child therapists to meet parents during the initial intake and find they are filled with fear or dread, asking questions like: "My child is constantly moving around and getting into trouble at school because he can't sit still in his seat…is that normal?" or "My daughter doesn't like to be alone and constantly needs attention…is that normal?" It is also not uncommon for child therapists to sit with parents and hear, during the initial intake, "Well…the domestic violence got really, really bad and she saw a lot of that happen but she was so little at the time…I've been told she won't remember it" or "He just seems so angry all the time, I don't know why he has become so angry, but I hear boys can be more aggressive than girls…is that normal?" We find ourselves in the position of shifting through narratives, observing parent and child behavioral patterns and collecting data to help us make determinations of what is considered normative and what may be considered atypical development prompting clinical diagnosis and care recommendations. Therapists do this while taking into consideration the cultural constructs making up a family system and specific memberships of majority or minority groups and communities. Child development encompasses several domains including physical, cognitive and emotional or social learning, all within the context of culture, microcultures and society.

Typical development can be organized into the following stages of developmental periods:

The prenatal period: from conception to birth

This period of development includes a rapid progression of life in which the vulnerability of life cannot be overstated either from the mother's viewpoint or the unborn child's (Slade *et al.* 2009).

Infancy and toddlerhood: birth to three years old

This is a three-year period in which the brain is continuing to rapidly develop and prune synaptic connections based on the environmental influences. During this phase of development there continue to be complex processes and children often use their senses to explore and understand the world (Ener 2016).

Early childhood: from three to six years old

Physical, social and cognitive development occurs in conjunction with physical growth and changes. Play serves as a means of supporting every aspect of psychological and physical development (Berk 2002).

Middle childhood: from six to eleven years old

Physical, social and cognitive development continues, and the context of school emerges, carrying new responsibilities and peer influences (Taylor and Workman 2018). Movement and play include participation in athletics or organized games, with rules and logic being hallmarks of this phase (Berk 2002).

An overview of developmental models
Gesell's maturational theory

Arnold Gesell, a key pioneer in child development in the early 1900s, hypothesized development occurs in a maturational manner, meaning in a specific order, when internal structures such as the heart, nervous system and motor functions are developing harmoniously alongside the individual's sociocultural environments (Gesell 1928). An infant who has discovered their feet will experience various means of sensorial interaction; for example, tactile and oral exploration of feet, the infant moving their own feet and/or passive exploration such as the infant's feet touching the ground, other individuals touching the infant's feet and feeling pain in their own feet. Maturational theory postulates this gradual awareness and mastery of the sensory experience cannot effectively progress without the prior successful development of the infant's nervous, motor and regulatory systems that allow the infant to engage in this process of movement and sensory exploration (Gesell 1928). Gesell postulated all development occurs in a cyclical, predictable manner, with each individual progressing through the sequence of development at their own pace. Within the cyclical process of development, the time between each stage of development increases with age, causing rapid development in infancy through adolescence and a slower cyclical process throughout early adulthood and later adulthood. Gesell's theory of maturational development laid the foundation for many developmental theories utilized in modern times to assess, explain and correct developmental deficits that may occur in children.

Erikson's psychosocial theory of development

Erik Erikson was a German developmental psychologist and psychoanalyst in the mid-1900s. Erikson's theory of psychosocial development suggests individuals progress through eight stages of development from birth to adulthood (Ray 2016). Erikson believed an individual's personality is shaped through their interactions with their culture, the people around them and their environments

(Shaffer 1999). Erikson's theory postulates that each stage presents the individual with a conflict which they must overcome to progress to the next stage of development (Ray 2016). Erikson believed children are active participants in their development and through this process they adapt, develop and build personality characteristics. For example, the first stage of Erikson's model, Trust versus Mistrust, takes place between infancy and 18 months of age. When presented with this conflict, the infant learns through daily caretaking whether their environment and caregivers are safe, stable and consistent enough to provide for the infant's basic needs (Shaffer 1999). Should the infant receive inconsistent or unstable caregiving, the infant begins to view their world as unsafe and untrustworthy (Shaffer 1999).

Erikson's psychosocial stages of development progress throughout an individual's life, presenting the individual with areas of mastery that pertain to developmental challenges such as trust, autonomy, self-esteem, confidence, identity formation, companionship, productivity and contentment with one's life choices and events (Shaffer 1999). It is important to note that Erikson was somewhat vague around how or why these stages of development occur and what might happen should an individual fail to progress through these stages (Shaffer 1999). Despite this ambiguity, Erikson's psychosocial theory of development is widely taught and utilized by a multitude of professions interested in social-emotional development.

Piaget's cognitive theory

Jean Piaget was a Swiss psychologist and epistemologist in the early and mid-1900s. Piaget's theory of cognitive development focuses on intellectual growth and development from birth to adolescence and beyond (Shaffer 1999). Like Erikson, Piaget believed development occurred in stages, with cognitive structures forming and progressing in complexity as a child takes an active role in learning to adapt to their environment. Piaget proposed five stages of cognitive development from birth to adolescence. The sensorimotor stage occurs from birth to two years of age and consists of an infant/young child utilizing their innate sensory and motor abilities to explore and subsequently learn about their environment. Initially, an infant's innate reflexes such as rooting, sucking, moro, grasping and stepping aid the infant in exploring their environment. As the infant masters the grasping reflex and learns to control higher order motor function, such as extending their arm, the infant learns to pair their grasping reflex with extending the arm to grab something within arm's reach. Piaget called these learning progressions "schemas" and posited that cognitive development builds upon existing schemas leading to greater complexity in cognitive capabilities. To utilize the example above, the infant now has a schema that informs the infant on how to reach and grasp something at arm's length. A likely subsequent developmental step within the sensorimotor stage may be the mastery of reaching, grasping and bending the arm to ultimately place the object into the infant's mouth, an activity that many parents find both adorable and maddening. Piaget's theory of cognitive development suggests development progresses in this structural manner as maturation and mastery of developmental tasks advance.

The preoperational stage of cognitive development follows the sensorimotor stage and takes place between ages two and seven years (Shaffer 1999). In the preoperational stage of development children engage in imaginative play and gradually understand that others may have a different perception of the world. The concrete operational stage occurs between ages seven and eleven and allows children to have a more logical, reality-based view of the world (Shaffer 1999). During this stage children are learning by observing the behaviors of others and inferring motivating factors behind these behaviors (Shaffer 1999). From eleven years of age and beyond individuals enter the formal operations stage of cognitive development, in which they can ponder abstract thought and apply logistical thinking and reasoning to hypothetical situations (Shaffer 1999). This aids the individual in problem solving and leads to the construction of executive functioning skills, such as thinking about consequences of one's actions prior to engaging in said action.

Piaget's cognitive theory led to an expansion in understanding within the field of developmental psychology and allowed researchers to build upon Piaget's theory to explore and construct additional developmental theories.

Vygotsky's cognitive development theory

Lev Vygotsky was a Soviet psychologist in the early 1900s whose cognitive development theory contributed to our understanding of early childhood development. Vygotsky's research provided extensive insight into the developmental processes that occur in young children. Vygotsky and colleagues used the term the *Zone of Proximal Development* to describe the potential for cognitive development in young children and the process through which children learn and master tasks. Vygotsky postulated that with the assistance of an adult or an individual with greater maturational abilities, a child can learn to master tasks beyond their "typical" developmental capabilities, or at the upper level of the Zone of Proximal Development. Additionally, Vygotsky postulated the lower level of the Zone of Proximal Development consists of a child exploring, learning and mastering tasks at a typically developing level. Vygotsky also shaped the concept of *scaffolding* or the difference between what a child can do with help and what a child cannot do without help. The concept of scaffolding is applied in multiple areas of child development such as psychotherapy, teaching, occupational therapy and early intervention. Furthermore, Vygotsky identified play as a vital mechanism in cognitive development for children, allowing children to engage in creative exploration in their natural environments, leading to development of problem solving skills and overall cognitive development (Ray 2016).

Kohlberg's moral development theory

Lawrence Kohlberg was an American psychologist in the mid–late 1900s whose theory suggests moral development takes place in stages similar to Piaget and Erikson's models. Kohlberg's theory consists of three levels and six stages starting in infancy and progressing to adulthood (Ray 2016). Kohlberg developed his theory by utilizing storytelling with children of different ages to examine how moral reasoning changed as children developed higher level cognitive function. Kohlberg was not interested in whether the children got the right answer, he focused more on the reasoning process utilized by the child to get their answer. Kohlberg followed the children he interviewed into adulthood at three-year intervals to examine and explore how reasoning changes with age. Kohlberg's efforts found children in the preconventional level of development, infancy through preschool ages, responded to the dilemmas in the stories with largely egocentric and individualistic reasoning. School-aged children (7–11 years) in Kohlberg's conventional level responded with more insight and knowledge around social currency and expectations within social relationships. Adolescents in the post-conventional level responded with an understanding of individuality, importance of familial relationships, basic human rights and a general understanding of legalities involved in each dilemma presented to them. Lastly, adults in the post-conventional level responded with a greater understanding of universal ethical principles and placed high value on acting in accordance with these principles (Ray 2016).

Kohlberg purported development through these stages took place as if on a ladder, where the child could only move forward through the stages and levels in the order listed, with each new stage replacing the reasoning skills of the previous stage. Additionally, Kohlberg suggested completion of all stages for every individual was not definite, with many individuals unable to apply a greater understanding of universal ethical principles to moral reasoning. Kohlberg's moral development theory is widely utilized today by professionals interested in child development and moral reasoning.

Greenspan's emotional development theory

Stanley Greenspan was an American child psychiatrist who built upon the theories of Piaget and Erikson but focused primarily on the emotional development of children. Greenspan researched and practiced in the 1970s through the 2000s. He studied the interplay between cognitive, social and emotional development and established theoretical building blocks of emotional development with six capacities or "milestones" essential to the foundation of learning and development throughout life. Each milestone builds upon the skills and abilities attained in the previous milestone, creating a scaffolded process of development. Greenspan's milestones of emotional development include: self-regulation, relations, communication, complex communication, abstract tho logical thought (Ray 2016). Greenspan believed children through these milestones by mastering challenges or conflicts to each capacity. Children who are unable to progress through a milestone require intervention to help correct their developmental trajectory and continue along the path of healthy emotional development.

Additionally, Greenspan highlighted the importance of "meeting children where they are" (Greenspan n.d.) within all areas of development to maximize the individualized potential for growth within each child. Greenspan created the "Greenspan Floortime Approach": an evidence-based early intervention technique which encourages and strengthens growth within the six milestone areas of emotional development for children with autism and other special needs. Greenspan's lifetime of research and practice contributed a wealth of knowledge to multiple professions interested in the field of early child development to include the Zero to Three movement, pediatrics, infant development and learning disorders. Zero to Three is a movement that began in the late 1970s to provide helpful tools and resources, practical policies and advocacy for early childhood development. The efforts of Zero to Three are to create influential change for parents, professionals and policy makers, thereby ensuring infants and toddlers have the strongest and best start in life (Zero to Three 2019).

It is important for professionals in a role of helping or advocating for children and families to have a solid understanding of developmental theory. Developmental theory is the foundation with which we begin to build the beliefs, values and viewpoints that guide our interests and decision-making within our professional practice. Knowledge regarding developmental theory is especially important in working with children and families who have experienced abuse, neglect or other forms of trauma, as we sometimes have the added role of advocate within court proceedings that often take place within family or criminal judicial arenas. A thorough understanding of developmental theory as it applies to the clients we work with is beneficial in presenting detailed testimony and quality advocacy for children and families.

Play therapy history, philosophy and practice
Early views of play

The eighteenth-century French philosopher Rousseau recognized the inherent value of play and games in child development. He was one of the first to advocate for studying the role of play to gain insight into children's behavior for providing appropriate education (Lebo 1955). He recommended that adults enter the child's world and participate in the play, because he considered play to be the gateway to understanding their thinking. Rousseau discussed his observations of how sensory and physical data received by children organizes their learning and thinking, creating outcomes related to their behavior. Rousseau explained that this occurs by the child having conscious or unconscious thoughts and sensations of what constitutes pleasant or unpleasant experiences in which they seek or avoid certain stimuli or objects as a result (Rousseau 1979). The body of research over the last several decades supports the phenomenon of learning occurring through experience, and defense mechanisms of avoidance of negative stimuli associated with trauma are hallmarks of post-traumatic stress (Van der Kolk 2014). Stress impacts imaginative play and many desirable educational outcomes, creative problem solving, development of sophisticated literacy and the development of socioemotional skills, including processing of complex ideas or information (Shuffelton 2012).

Play environments as a grounding principle

Play supports the developmental and emotional needs of children and is considered so important that it is recognized as optimizing the social emotional health and functioning of a child; therefore play has been recognized by the United Nations High Commission for Human Rights as a right for every child (Ginsburg 2007; Landreth 1991).

Axline (1969) demonstrated that play is the child's natural medium for self-expression. Children can express a wide range of emotions and cognitions through their play and play is considered the most appropriate mode of processing experiences for healing. Play captures a child's interest and intellectual creativity (Carey, Zaitchik and Bascandziev 2015; Findling, Bratton and Henson 2006; Henderson and Thompson 2015). When a child is offered the option of playing out their feelings or problems, just as they are, within the context of a relationship which holds unconditional positive regard, empathic understanding and authenticity, they can have an experience similar to what we may consider as support in adult therapy.

Play aids in children identifying what risks can be taken and how to modulate their affect in order to engage in decision-making. Almon (2017) describes the example of an adult driver engaging in risk analysis as they enter a stream of moving traffic: Is the gap large enough for me? Is what I'm driving fast enough? All the while, the adult driver is managing their breathing rates and modulating affect with the mind and body to organize around the stress, which is dependent upon their biological make-up and how past experiences have shaped them. Children in play face similar issues: Am I strong enough to climb that tree? Will those limbs hold me? All the while, the child is managing breathing rates and modulating affect with the mind and body to organize around the stress, which is dependent upon their biological make-up and how experiences have shaped them. These childhood experiences impact future experiences as an adult. When we begin conversations about how adverse childhood experiences impact the body, let's keep in mind how all experiences assist in shaping who we are.

The importance of creating space for creativity and play to promote thinking is highlighted in the literature about the life of Albert Einstein. He had to hire a scribe to take notes for his classes, enabling him to skip school to escape boredom, as a traditional classroom environment did not allow for free movement and person-centered play and learning (Lillard 2005). Maria Montessori saw the need for creativity and positive emotional climates to support powerful learning and proposed a radical shift within our education system during the early twentieth century. She created the "prepared environment" that motivated students to acquire new knowledge, and observed and documented how the optimal space paired with a warm relationship could connect a child with expansive and integrated thinking (Montessori 2014). The concept of a "Children's House" was created as an emblem based on Raphael's "Madonna della Seggiola." Raphael represented universal social progress and elevation of the idea of caring through depiction of a woman protecting her offspring alongside a figure of St. John, who represented humanity (Montessori 2014; Thoenes 2016). Montessori considered a secure space designed for children to be a basic human right. Montessori principles, echoed by the play therapy community, include multi-sensory experiences embedded within an environment of safety as fundamental in creating the ability for children to learn and grow. Professional adaptation of the environment to meet the unique and specific needs for the child is fundamental. Understanding the best methodology for learning supports our ability to expand these ideas to therapy and emotional or behavioral processing. Play therapy creates a similar environment to that outlined by Maria Montessori. It combines developmentally informed child-centered multi-sensory processing and utilizes the philosophy of Rousseau for entering the child's world through play. Imaginative play activities provide intellectual, social and emotional benefits for children (Soundy 2009). Carefully designed child-sized environments provide encouragement for independence and autonomy, enabling children to approach their reality through a personal voyage of discovery embedded in sensory experiences, practical activities and supportive relationships (Soundy 2009).

Developmental progression of play

The concept of play is not a new idea. Greek philosopher Plato, in his *Laws*, voices that play creates opportunity for children's learning and play supports a child's character; play needs to include continual physical movement with music, dance or gymnastics combined within the play in order for children to grow and achieve mastery

(Bury 1961). Lev Vygotsky investigated play and suggested ways in which adults could help children use play symbolically, believing that children's play fostered spontaneous concepts and that play offered children the ability to take on various roles and perspectives within learning self-regulation (Bergen 2015).

Children's play aligns developmentally with their social, emotional, cognitive and physical growth following various stages of development. This is seen within Mildred Parten's influential research identifying the development of children's play and continues to be a reference for researchers and therapists alike in identifying normative play patterns or behaviors. Again, we emphasize the importance of overlaying cultural characteristics and considerations to any play assessment building upon this foundational work. Parten's work includes stages of development within play that are broken down into six distinct styles (Frost, Wortham and Reifel 2011; Grote-Garcia *et al.* 2017):

Unoccupied play: Children do not play with others, instead they occupy themselves with other tasks (e.g. looking around the room).

Solitary play: Children play alone with their own toys. Independent work is seen with very little interaction with others. Typically, this is seen between birth to two years of age.

Parallel play: Includes children continuing to play on their own. This play can occur alongside other children who may or may not be using similar toys or the same toys as the other child. This type of play is most typically seen at ages two to three.

Associative play: Children are beginning to play with others, sharing toys and often following a storyline. Associative play behaviors are seen between four to five and a half years of age.

Cooperative play: This is considered one of the highest levels of social play, where children play in groups and everyone is cooperating to achieve common goals. This play involves children having the ability to negotiate with one another and hosts the phenomenon of children assuming "roles" within the play, taking turns and making suggestions within negotiations about changing the storyline or plot. Play which includes games and rules is considered a part or aspect of cooperative play involving winners and losers. The games often have child-controlled rules and may have strict rules such as seen within sports or athletics. This play typically appears by age six and continues throughout life.

Onlooker play: When a child watches another child playing but makes no attempt to join in. This type of play can be seen throughout life.

Developmental progression of children's art

Children's art also follows various stages of development depending upon the child's age and developmental period of life, with influences from the family system and children's culture. There are sociocultural influences which impact the motivation to draw or attitudes towards art in general. Culture influences the content of children's art expressions (Malchiodi 1998) including race, gender identities, sexuality in the family system, socioeconomic status, regional or geographic location, ethnicity, citizenship and community systems. There are also considerations with family or cultural norms and what may be taught within the home as a value system around making a mess. Some children will struggle with spontaneous or child-directed work because there is an expectation of adult authority or the therapist being in a teaching role. Messy art may create anxiety as family norms or values dictate cleanliness and respect for being a guest in another person's environment. Part of our work includes helping manage and control mess during creative expression while allowing the child freedom to make a mess. Play and expressive arts therapists are talented human beings!

Rubin (2005, p.35) discusses stages within the developmental art process to include "manipulating, forming, naming, representing, containing, experimenting, consolidating, naturalizing, personalizing."

The following stages of children's art development are adapted from Rubin (2005):

Manipulating (one to two years) includes the first stage and encounter with materials to manipulate either appropriately or inappropriately. The behaviors are not inappropriate to the toddler but defined by the environment. Sensory qualities of materials are important, including texture, kinesthetic movement and tension.

Forming (two to three years) centers on children gaining control over movements as they begin to make more deliberate actions regarding what happens with art materials. Children may practice art and repeat motions or activities such as circular scribbling, rolling or flattening of Play-Doh and clay. Shapes may form within the art as a precursor to intentional forms.

Naming (three to four years) consists of the child naming their creation. Rubin hypothesizes this could result from adults wanting to know what has been made. Human figures are simple, including shapes that have a head and body but which become limited on extensions or facial details. Children may experiment as they did in their early representational phase, but in a way similar to manipulative exploration. They explore through making and creating, testing freedom and flexibility and finding delight in demonstrating ability to create mass within human drawings and fill in the lines.

Representing (four to six years) includes a time when true representations occur from the manipulating, forming and naming process. These representations may appear odd to adult eyes but make sense in the eyes of a child. Work often includes what is of interest to children and they continue to practice different ways of doing or making various items. Experimentation includes beginning representations of human figures having a head–body with extensions towards more solid creations of human figures by the end of this developmental period.

Consolidating (six to nine years) occurs as children find preferred ways of communicating pictorially. Schematic views for how the world works emerge within their artwork and pictures take realistic shape and can include movement (catching of a ball, running, flying, etc.). Pictures can begin to uncover "what lies beneath", meaning children will begin to draw what is underground or within the water or an x-ray into the human body, capturing a layered quality of understanding for the world around or within them.

Naturalizing (nine to twelve years) depicts increasing elaboration and sophistication in nonfigurative work. Art is more proportional, includes more landscapes and has increased spatial relationships. Emotion is reflected in more complex tones and children become more self-critical of their own work.

Personalizing (twelve to eighteen years) includes the period of naturalizing, moving forward throughout late grade school and into early adolescence. The art process becomes active and children may engage with multiple forms of media with increased control. Self-criticism and concern about quality increases with comparisons to other art within a social context. Art can take on an abstract quality as cognition matures enhancing creativity and symbolic meaning.

Art within mental health settings is an active process facilitated within the therapeutic context. Children who present as anxious, hyperactive or emotionally overwhelmed can quickly engage in chaotic discharge, particularly if the materials are not carefully chosen by the therapist (Malchiodi 1998). Materials that need more time and control or could result in regression (messy materials such as wet paint) may benefit from being placed in a location out of reach for small hands, to ensure this type of art material is prepared and supported by the therapist's limit-setting. Materials which have ease of use, such as loose paper, colored pencils, crayons or pastels and markers, can be placed on lower shelves to support freedom of expression.

The use of art materials in session is a process for play therapists. Art, similarly to play, can be implemented from a variety of theoretical perspectives. Depending upon the therapist's theoretical orientation or goal within the session, art can be used to enhance the therapeutic process. The product or result of art-making is only one factor. Expressive therapists pay close attention to the process of art-making. This includes the level of frustration a child experiences, self-criticism, forming of objects, whether they are sculptures, paintings or drawings, level of intensity or focus and relational qualities within the creation itself and between the child and therapist. The information received provides data to the therapist regarding the child's inner world of emotions, cognitions and perception of self in relation to the environment.

Early pioneers in psychotherapy play applications

Freud first discussed the concept of repetitious thinking patterns and behaviors, describing the phenomenon as being related to unconscious conflict within the mind and the defense mechanism of repression designed to serve us by keeping memories hidden (Freud 1896). Freud was also first to offer the approach of therapy with individuals who had experienced trauma by offering multiple methods of allowing memories to emerge. He opened the world to the impact trauma has on adult lives, which prompted exploration of child psychology. Freud engaged in the first attempt of child therapy with Little Hans in an effort to alleviate a phobia anxiety response (Freud 1963). Direct observation of children was among the first techniques adopted by child psychoanalysts beginning the movement towards play therapy.

Hermine Hug-Hellmuth is cited as being one of the first professionals to record direct observations of play, and presented a paper to the Psychoanalytic Society in 1913 (Johnson 2015). She drew theoretical conclusions from the play behaviors, although she did not adopt Rousseau's framework of entering into the world of play as a full participant. Her approach included more of an ethnographic study to better understand human development and the phenomenology of the child.

Melanie Klein was initially inspired by Freud and formulated psychological principles of infant analysis in 1927 (Lebo 1955). She differed from the psychoanalytic community and Hug-Hellmuth as her thoughts and theories moved towards children having capacity for insight (Berzoff 2016). She named her model psychoanalytic play technique, or play analysis, and found the best toys to conduct such analysis were small and simple, thus allowing children to project their own meaning onto the toys (Klein 1955). Klein was the first to share her interpretations with the children she worked with using their expressions, symbols or metaphors in the context of what was being played out. She believed in the power of play and how it provided an outlet for expressing what the child viewed as unacceptable wishes or feelings (Johnson 2015). Klein states: "In interpreting not only the child's words but also his activities with his toys, I applied this basic principle to the mind of the child, whose play and varied activities, in fact his whole behavior, are means of expressing what the adult expresses predominantly by words" (1955, p.4).

Anna Freud was another psychoanalyst to contribute to the development of play therapy. Her career included a substantial focus on assessment and the necessity of appropriate training in child psychology to correctly understand the etiology of concerns. Anna Freud was the first to suggest making use of a wider scope of data, including observations of the child by the analyst in unstructured play sessions, structured assessments of the child including cognitive assessments or projective testing, diagnostic interviews with parents, reports from the school and any other relevant information to conclude assessments and clinical formulation (Midgley 2011). Much of Anna Freud's work used child's play in an analogous way to the work with adults and dreams (Lebo 1955). She went against the trend of her day, pioneering the importance of diagnosis, not simply as centered around symptom clusters for children, but to regard the age and developmental phase of the child. She argued symptoms in childhood can be transitory and have many different meanings at different times of the lifespan (Abrams 2001; Midgley 2011). All early clinicians within the field of child psychotherapy and analysis stressed the emotional relationship between the child and therapist.

Present-day knowledge of play therapy philosophy to counter-condition adversity

Play is the natural language of the child and thought of as the easiest way for children to express troubling thoughts and feelings from both the conscious and unconscious mind (Drewes and Schaefer 2014).

Ginsburg (2007) states that "play is essential to child development because it contributes to the cognitive, physical, social and emotional well-being of children and youth" (p.182). Play provides balance and safety due to the symbolic nature of materials and child expression (Landreth 2001; Shelan and Stewart 2015); creative arts, including play practices, have a unique role in the treatment of trauma for those who have difficulty with verbal expression (Malchiodi 2008). However, there is a concern across disciplines including education, pediatric medicine, occupational therapy and mental health regarding free play being markedly reduced within young lives for many children (Ginsburg 2007; Louv 2008; O'Brien and Smith 2002). For young trauma survivors with limited language, or those who may be unable to put experiences into words, play offers a means of communicating ideas without words and can be hypothesized as a protective factor for childhood development.

Play in the context of therapy

Play therapy of itself is not a theory, but an application or way of putting theory into practice. Yalom (2002) discusses therapeutic factors as the actual mechanisms which create change, and this is reflected within the play therapy principles highlighted in Drewes and Schaefer (2014) discussing the therapeutic powers of play. "Therapeutic powers transcend culture, language, age and gender... therapeutic powers of play refer to the specific change agents in which play initiates, facilitates or strengthens their therapeutic effect" (Drewes and Schaefer 2014, pp.1–2). There is no one central definition of play; however, researchers often describe play as holding several distinct properties including: being pleasurable or enjoyable, having no extrinsic goals (done for its own sake), including freedom from time, embodying a diminished consciousness of the self, being spontaneous and voluntary with active engagement and having imagination or make-believe qualities (Brown 2010; Ray 2011). Almon (2017, p.2) writes about how the Playwork Principles Security Group defines play:

Play is a process which is freely chosen, personally directed and intrinsically motivated. That is, children and young people determine and control the content and intent of their play, by following their own instincts, ideas and interests in their own way for their own reasons.

These play definitions highlight the consistent principles of allowing children to take the lead and direct their own work, which is a founding principle of child-centered play therapy. However, play therapy is not always fun or pleasurable and many children enter the play therapy room angry, sad, grieving, fearful and/or engaged in play behaviors we may interpret as repetitious and lacking all joy, holding a trauma experience in a state of reenactment (Terr 1990). Many theorists, researchers and clinicians describe how trauma experiences are quickly incorporated into the mind and body, derived from a state of helplessness, which can be projected onto relationships or through actions and behaviors such as play (Ford and Cloitre 2009; Karr-Morse and Wiley 2012; Levine 1997; Siegel 2003; Terr 1990; Van der Kolk 2014; Van der Kolk and McFarlane 1996). Eliana Gil (2006) discusses play within the context of child trauma, building upon and refining Terr's original construct of "post-traumatic play." Post-traumatic play described by Gil is a stylized form of play with unique characteristics including its repetitive, literal and highly structured nature (Gil 2006). Terr (1990) states "as opposed to ordinary child's play, post-traumatic play is obsessively repeated. It is grim" (p.239). Gil echoes this, voicing that children are engrossed with the trauma reenactment play, in which energy shifts and the common features of the play begin to wane. Children appear to play in such a way that it lacks spontaneity, laughter (or laughter appears incongruent) and pretend, or role play simply doesn't appear (Gil 2006). Terr emphasizes the dangers of post-traumatic play within her research. This is confirmed and acknowledged by Gil; however, she also voices the potential benefits of a child's self-imposed gradual exposure to the trauma content through play and that the play itself may be an attempt to desensitize the feared stimulus or adverse experience, allowing for mastery to be achieved (Gil 2006). Play can provide the protective space or cushion, allowing children the ability to distance themselves from trauma content or adverse experiences within memories while simultaneously externalizing them in a manner that titrates the experience in a tolerable way (Gil 2017).

Play therapy: advancing definitions

The definition of play including pleasure or enjoyment has been discussed by Vygotsky and within Maria Montessori's (2014) writings. Play is further defined within the context of trauma in the research of both Terr (1990) and Gil (2006). Ray (2011) draws upon play research and includes the argument for the need to expand our definitions of play by describing the nuances of play. These nuances include therapeutic play in the context of trauma, meaning how play may encompass games and activities in which a child does not always derive pleasure. Therefore, play therapy is better described as an activity in which the child is free from adult direction, actively engaged, experiencing flow with little self-consciousness and has the opportunity to be released from literal grounding in reality. Guiding this play therapy principle is a person-centered, or a humanistic theoretical, base that draws upon early pioneers such as Carl Rogers and Virginia Axline. Play therapy can also be defined to include cognitive principles and adult directed activities. This framework posits the therapist taking the lead in therapy and setting goal-directed play or art-based activities which bring any number of theories into practice. The central framework of either approach is that play is the natural medium in which children can express thoughts, emotions and experiences. Toys can become words and clinicians adequately trained in play therapy have the unique position of being able to translate play into narratives that support the overall integration of adversity and trauma.

Therapeutic art

Offering the child an ability to engage in creative expression may come in the form of art including sculpture, painting, movement, photography, drawing or using other forms of art media to create representations of their experience and sense of self. The American Art Therapy Association (2013, p.1) description includes:

> Art therapy is a mental health profession in which clients, facilitated by the art therapist, use art media, the creative process and the resulting artwork to explore their feelings, reconcile emotional conflicts, foster self-awareness, manage behavior and addictions, develop social skills, improve reality orientation, reduce anxiety and increase self-esteem. A goal in art therapy is to improve or restore a client's functioning and his or her sense of personal well-being. Art therapy practice requires knowledge of visual art (drawing, painting, sculpture and other art forms) and the creative process.

Creative arts therapists or play therapists do not seek to interpret the work but instead allow the child to discover their own personal meaning within the process. The training and comprehensive degree program for art therapy warrants respect and clear understanding that a play therapist can utilize art therapeutically, but they should not refer to themselves as an "art therapist" without the degree, licensing or credentialing. Many play therapists will use drawings, painting, sculpture or prop-based art activities to support children in their work, often as an adjunct to other play activities (Malchiodi 1998). The activity can be purposeful, which directs children to draw, paint or create a project that represents a treatment goal or objective the therapist is seeking to meet, or the activity can be open to the child's creativity. The child-centered approach offers opportunity for spontaneity within creation and design. Play therapists view children's art as non-verbal expression similar to play and these graphic representations of the thought or emotional process can enhance the play therapy process (Malchiodi 1998).

The child may or may not explain in words the meaning of the art; however, therapists pay close attention to the process of how the work was created, noting body language, intensity and any verbalizations or specific emphasis the child places upon the work. Expressive arts therapists and play therapists can use verbal techniques for helping children explore perceptions rather than moving towards a role of interpretation (Malchiodi 2008). Art can offer a means of communication for creative growth which transcends language an provides the ability for a child to put into words through images what couldn't be said.

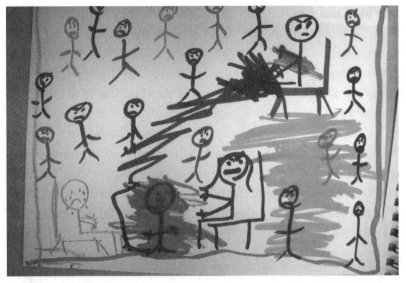

Figure 1.1 A therapeutic art picture drawn by a young boy using markers. The referral was prompted due to the client's diagnosis of selective mutism; however, without any use of words he created this image to represent his family system

The co-authors of this text utilize art through non-directive and directive approaches within the play therapy process and utilize art through movement within yoga practice to allow children the opportunity to sculpt using their body and/or movements for creating a narrative or representation of self, thought or feeling. We utilize traditional art materials as a means of integrating content. This process allows for us to shift thinking away from repetitive patterns by incorporating new sensory experiences into the mind, body and therapeutic relationship.

Play therapy and art in clinical practice

Play therapy within clinical practice can often take the form of direct or non-direct practice. Directive and non-directive play therapy very much as they sound. Directive work assumes f the therapist taking the lead and organizing the rocess in a manner which supports the overarching ssion and treatment plan in general. The process pecific tasks or the therapist may move the session in one direction or another depending on the decisions they make regarding reflection statements. The purpose of reflection can access unconscious thoughts or influence the child. Non-directive play therapy practices have the approach of the child taking the lead and the therapist not structuring the session. Therapists reflect content or thematic qualities of the play or relationship factors in a manner that does not necessarily intervene to the point in which the therapist is now driving the direction of the session. Most typically, non-directive child-centered play therapy is grounded within a client-centered and humanistic theoretical framework, while directive play therapy practices can include cognitive behavioral work, solution-focused interventions (Berg and Steiner 2003), Theraplay® (Booth and Jernberg 2009), Gestalt (Oaklander 1988), ecosystemic play therapy (O'Connor 2000), Adlerian (Kottman 2001), prescriptive play therapy (Schaefer 2011) or narrative theories, to name a few types of theoretical approaches for application of play. The therapist draws upon their stylistic theory to guide the session or treatment tasks. We (Michelle and Lindsay) advocate for an integrated approach to working with children impacted by adversity and stress by drawing upon the necessary theories (those of which a therapist has mastery and therefore lie within their scope of practice) and a strong knowledge base of neurobiology to conceptualize the presenting issues, formulate ideas regarding diagnosis and develop a treatment plan that is intentional and prescriptive to the unique needs of the child or family system.

CHAPTER 2

The Mind–Body Connection

YOGA AND PLAY TO ADDRESS ADVERSE EXPERIENCES FOR CHILDREN

Defining adverse childhood experiences (ACEs)

Kelly arrived for her first play therapy session hearing from her parent, "This is your special feelings doctor, don't just play the whole time, talk about the things you need to! I hope you have fun!" What a contradictory idea for a child? Don't play, instead talk about your terrible experiences, yet have fun. Kelly understood she needed to talk and that she was expected to talk about what she had seen and experienced at home with a stranger she had just met, yet this supposedly would be fun? A confusing experience indeed and one which is common for children who have experienced maltreatment and multiple experiences of adversity. Kelly wasn't a novice to therapy and the first session included a child who was terrified to enter another provider's office and who didn't want to talk about what had happened to her. She didn't look at all like fun was an expected result for this new experience as she solemnly walked down the hall towards the playroom with her head down and shoulders slumped.

Felitti and colleagues (1998) published a study on adverse childhood experiences (ACEs), initiating a conversation about early childhood exposure to abuse and the long-term health implications. The original ACE questionnaire included a sample of participants insured by Kaiser Permanente and described seven categories of ACEs: three categories focused on child maltreatment (exposure to physical abuse, sexual abuse, psychological abuse/neglect) and four categories focused on household dysfunction (divorce, incarceration, maternal or paternal mental health illness, domestic violence) with a total score spanning all seven categories on the measure yielding a score between zero and ten. The original study was developed utilizing a sample of predominantly white, upper middle-class individuals. Criticism regarding question structure has been fair. Questions are not inclusive to all gender identities and experiences. Categorizations of domestic violence through adverse childhood experiences research typically specify a child witnessing the abuse of their mother; however, this limitation of gender excludes the possibility of an individual identifying as male having experienced abuse or violence. Given our understanding of disparities within communities and larger societal systems, it is imperative we also take a closer look at the theoretical concept of intersectionality and broaden our thinking around what constitutes an ACE to include factors associated with marginalization, oppression, poverty and how the intersection of identity, including race, gender or spiritual ideological associations, impacts health outcomes. Qualitative data provides evidence that race, unsafe neighborhoods, community violence, bullying and experiences within the foster care system are all significant factors in adversity and poor health outcomes (Cronholm *et al.* 2015). Furthermore, Sue and Sue (2016) highlight that adverse experiences can be expanded to include environmental "injustices," which include dirty industries and other pollution-producing operations frequently located in urban and rural areas where people of lower socioeconomic status or people of color live. We are beginning to understand the physiological pathways adversity brings to a life, including cognitive and physical impairment in addition to high risk behaviors (Cronholm *et al.* 2015), and expanding our thinking from classification within groups to include the richer complexity of the human experience within intersectionality means redefining how we view ACEs.

Kelly began life by experiencing the effects of intimate partner violence in utero. We understand that intimate partner violence (IPV) during the time of pregnancy can lead to devastating consequences. This may encompass, for mothers, physical in depression and post-traumatic symptoms. Infants can experienc birth weight, small gestational age, reduced head circumference and chronic stress hormones that impact sensitive developing systems (Cha and Masho 2014; Peña, Monk and Champagne 2012). Research links the effects of IPV in utero to adverse outcomes, including increased levels of cortisol and corticotrophin-releasing hormone in the mother and fetus which alter the programming of fetal neurons and subsequently impact child behavior later in life (Flach *et al.* 2011). Increases in maternal cortisol can also create fetal overexposure to glucocorticoids, which are associated with anxiety and stress, crossing the placenta into the fetal environment (Glover 2016). Glucocorticoids are steroid hormones secreted by the adrenal gland and associated with the stress response within the sympathetic nervous system (Sapolsky 1994). IPV is not only linked to increased stress, but to postpartum depression, which impacts mother–infant attachment and may lead to adverse child development (Flach *et al.* 2011).

During pregnancy, Kelly's family also faced significant financial difficulties due to the loss of her father's job. Allegations of inappropriate touching of students were voiced, which prompted a leave of absence and subsequent loss of her father's teaching position, leading to a change in career to contracting in the construction industry. Kelly's mother struggled with IPV within the home for years, including emotional abuse and physical altercations. They faced significant financial distress as Kelly's father attempted to find work while she stayed at home to care for the infant. The legal system became involved to investigate allegations of potential child abuse within the educational system in which he had worked, resulting in financial strain to account for legal defense funds.

Kelly was diagnosed at age four with a sensory processing disorder. The physician raised concerns about Kelly's development in bilateral coordination, fine motor coordination, gross motor skills, posture and core strength, visual motor skills and sensory overwhelm. Kelly began treatment with an occupational therapist to improve functioning and sensory integration. The occupational therapist noted Kelly's difficulty in regulating her arousal level so it often seemed greatly out of sync with the activity or task; for example, she would experience "meltdowns" that might not immediately make sense to the observor in relation to its trigger. These meltdowns were a result of her the inability to self-regulate her emotions, which was a significant concern. Sensory modulation or the ability to regulate and organize reactions to sensory input in a graded and adaptive manner was compromised. She demonstrated to her occupational therapist difficulties in modulating tactile input, sensitivity to light or unexpected touch and certain self-care routines such as brushing her teeth or bathing. Kelly struggled with vestibular or proprioception modulation, which impacted her orientation of body in space and responses to multi-sensory inputs.

The year Kelly turned five, her mother finalized a long, high-conflict divorce which had enveloped her in a state of fear of her partner and distrust in the system. The court system did not find sufficient evidence of violence or a threat of harm and the parents were awarded shared custody. Kelly's mother left the relationship and attempted to share parenting time of Kelly. This resulted in further complications as the couple was unable to co-parent effectively due to the ongoing conflict, fear, suspicion and need for control. There were multiple exhausting court experiences, all constituted as high conflict, with Kelly caught in the middle.

There is a significant body of research demonstrating the impact of divorce on family systems, including long-term health implications (Anda *et al.* 2006). It is further recognized by the courts that divorce impacts children negatively, with issues including adjustment problems, chronic stress, poverty due to changing economics, behavioral conduct issues, academic decline and disruption within parental relationship and attachment (Ferraro *et al.* 2016). Therefore, divorce education programs are designed and offered to help prevent co-parenting problems and provide children with a psychoeducational support group to process the impact of divorce. Kelly's family was referred to the local children's divorce program, which resulted in a poor outcome. As the divorce unfolded and custody arrangements were finalized, the process had taken a toll on the entire family.

Kelly displayed intense behaviors including aggression, anger and inconsolable "tantrums." Neither parent could be in the same room with the other, therefore were trying to find separate times to attend the program. Kelly was required to attend classes by the court; she left group sessions dysregulated and oscillating between intense anger and intense sadness until she collapsed, falling asleep in tears.

Kelly's mother was accepted into a graduate program for art education and relocated to another state to attend school in an attempt to better her life and set herself and her child up for success long term following the divorce. She was unable to bring Kelly as relocation of the minor out of state was not a possibility within the divorce decree. Kelly lived with her father during the program and her mother visited as much as possible, about once every few months. Kelly was able to travel out of state and would stay with her mother a couple of times per year. However, the abrupt change in circumstances resulted in loss for Kelly. She experienced a grief response associated with the loss of her primary attachment figure. Coupled with chronic stress, fear and violence, Kelly was left in a world of uncertainty.

Attachment as a fundamental principle

Attachment behaviors are thought to be borrowed from the behavioral concept of ethology to describe a system that leads to predictable outcomes, all of which contribute to survival of the species (Cassidy 2008). Knowledge of attachment theory paired with appropriate psychotherapy can promote neural integration and recovery (Siegel 2003). Conceptually, attachment behaviors include the central notion that there may be several different behaviors organized within the individual response to internal and external cues (Bowlby 1969) and these cues are a derivative of the stress response system to alert the individual when it is necessary to seek a secure base. Attachment is theorized to be a system in which the child is far from being a tabula rasa at birth, but rather equipped with the necessary mechanism to become activated when threatened. Attentive caregiving soothes, organizes and sustains interpersonal connectedness (Badenoch 2008; Bowlby 1969). From an evolutionary perspective, attachment is adaptive and necessary for child survival. It is also common for the attachment behavior of a child to mirror that of their caregiver. The attachment research provides support that 85 percent of the time a child's attachment experience in life in general will parallel the working model of attachment to the primary caregiver (Hesse 2008; Hesse and Main 2000).

The attachment system becomes disrupted with trauma, separation and loss. Research in animal studies documented by Harry Harlow with rhesus infant monkeys provides some insight into the innate systems with which an organism is born. Observations were made at intervals during a three-week period of separation between an infant monkey and its mother (Bowlby 1976). Although the infant monkey had contact with a sibling, it displayed little interest and play behavior and often sat in isolation; when provided a visual view of its mother it engaged in violent and prolonged protest with high-pitched screeching, crying and numerous attempts at hurling itself at the cage. The monkey infants became clingy with their mothers when reunited and ensured contact always throughout the day and night; researchers concluded the behavior was to avoid further separation (Bowlby 1976). Separation of an infant or child from a primary attachment figure creates a significant distress response seen not only in animal studies, but in human infant studies. Mary Ainsworth developed the "strange situation" to measure mother–child attachment behavior systems and patterns and this is widely used in attachment theory research. She demonstrated that children became anxious and distressed upon separation from a mother and the resulting observation of the system, primarily upon reunion from separation, yielded the quality of the attachment relationship (Van Rosmalen, Van der Veer and Van der Horst 2015). These early bonds and attachment styles include secure, insecure and disorganized attachment, which create the foundation of affect regulation with future relationships within adulthood through neural wiring of the brain (Badenoch 2008).

The left hemisphere of the brain functions to interpret relationships and environmental data, searching for the cause-effect. This occurs in a linear, logical mode of cognition, while the right hemisphere holds mediate autonoetic consciousness and autobiographical memory incorporating social cognition and theory of mind (Siegel 2003). The human ability to mentally place oneself in the past, in the present and in the future, or in counterfactual situations, thus to be able to examine our own thoughts, is considered an autonoetic consciousness. Research supports the idea that securely attached children have more enhanced emotional flexibility, can self-regulate during times of distress, have a more integrated narrative and achieve stable autonoetic consciousness, engage socially in a more functional manner and show resilience in the future when facing adversity (Siegel 2003). Divorce and parental separation are recognized as an adverse childhood experience (ACE) which disrupts attachment bonds and creates an activated stress response.

Kelly experienced exposure to IPV during prenatal development and throughout early childhood, and experienced both high conflict divorce and parental separation with her primary attachment figure, resulting in significant dysregulation and attachment rupture. Attachment does have a biological and evolutionary purpose; however, it is the subjective experience of the social interaction between the caregiver and the infant which maintains the bond (Anderson and Gedo 2013; Benedict 2006; Mercer 2006; Silverman 1998). The social interactions Kelly absorbed included violence, separation, grief and loss, uncertainty, confusion and instability.

Adverse experiences create disruption in development

Kelly's behaviors and "meltdowns" increased in frequency, duration and intensity, prompting a referral by a pediatrician to behavioral health services where she began parent–child interaction therapy (PCIT). Kelly began PCIT with both parents at a local behavioral health clinic which specialized in child and adolescent mental health. PCIT is an evidence-based treatment for working with parents and young children in which the therapist can help coach parents during real-time interactions (McNeil and Hembree-Kigin 2011). Most often this is done through a one-way mirror in which the parent has a "bug" in the ear to listen to therapist prompts. This helps remove the therapist from the actual physical interaction between parent and child. During child-directed interactions, parents learn and use play therapy skills to enhance their relationship. During parent-directed interactions, parents learn and use skills to improve child compliance, thus decreasing problem behaviors (McNeil and Hembree-Kigin 2011). The goal of Kelly's treatment was to reduce tantrums and behavioral outbursts as well as to help both parents find new ways to parent more effectively and improve parent–child relationships and child compliance. These services were ended after a few months when the family was determined to be unable to meet the requirements for treatment regimens. Kelly's parents had difficulty attending appointments regularly, with Kelly's mother trying to travel from out of state and her father working; Kelly struggled within the program, often screaming and yelling from the car to the waiting room that she didn't want to go to therapy.

When Kelly turned six, her mother graduated and returned home. Kelly resumed a traditional shared parenting plan, moving back and forth between two homes. Kelly's mother was unable to find work and they lived with Kelly's grandmother in tight living quarters. Resources were scarce as her mother struggled financially to make ends meet. That summer, Kelly and her father went on a camping trip with her grandfather who was mauled and killed by a bear, which then escaped back into the woods. Kelly began to complain of somatic issues, experienced frequent urinary infections, struggled with sleep, digestion, encopresis, enuresis and headaches. She began smearing feces while at school and melted down in the classroom throughout the day, was aggressive with peers, impulsive and struggled to pay attention, often not following directions from teachers or other authority figures, resulting in multiple visits to the pediatrician and other specialists.

Kelly was exhibiting such extreme behavioral issues following the summer that it prompted her next experience with mental health services. Kelly entered another behavioral-based program for PCIT. Kelly's mother engaged in a two-hour intake with Kelly at her side. During that time, she was asked to recount the entire history in detail. Kelly was noted by the therapist to be nervous and anxious during the intake session, which was evidenced by her standing close to her mother, lying on her mother's lap and trying to get in between the therapist and her mother to give her mother kisses. She was noted by the therapist to often grasp at her mother's face, pulling her hair or poking at her for attention. The therapist documented that Kelly struggled to take her own seat, to sit still and that she didn't approach the shelves of toys even once, which was flagged as being unusual and atypical for her developmental age. Kelly was described as feeling uncomfortable and embarrassed about her recent behaviors, as she would only whisper answers to the therapist's questions in her mother's ear. Kelly received a diagnosis of attention deficit hyperactivity disorder, separation anxiety disorder and was also identified as having delays in speech and motor functioning. She was referred back to occupational therapy and speech language therapy for treatment.

Kelly struggled at school both academically and socially with peers. She was described as "spacey," "difficult," and she challenged directions or transitions among activities. Kelly began smearing feces in the bathroom and was recorded by her teachers as lying about the incidents to avoid getting in trouble. PCIT began in which Kelly verbally protested going to therapy in addition to throwing tantrums prior to and following sessions. The experience included another discharge prior to the completion of treatment as Kelly was considered "non-compliant" with her care. The school continued to urge Kelly's mother to seek treatment and voiced that, without a change in behavior, they would not be able to continue to support Kelly within the school and might need to expel her for ongoing disruptions and vandalism to school property.

Kelly connected to play therapy nearing age seven after having exposure to multiple adverse life experiences since infancy. I began to organize her case, focusing on a formulation which included high levels of adverse childhood experiences and trauma. Exposure to adversity coupled with chronic poverty, disrupted attachment, complex family systems and legal systems were all possible explanations for disorganized thinking patterns. Her subsequent behavior problems stemmed from a dysregulated nervous system.

The concept of the original work on ACEs continues to be reviewed. Findings by researchers solidify the importance and understanding that the effects of early childhood trauma on the developing brain and nervous system are critical. Health outcomes associated with increasing numbers of adverse experiences or trauma experiences are consistent, including chronic stress, substance use and abuse, behavioral issues, poor work performance, self-esteem deficits, anxiety, depression, learning deficits and emotional regulation deficiencies. Projected long-term risks for chronic disease include illnesses such as liver disease, ischemic heart disease, chronic obstructive pulmonary disease (COPD) and premature death (Anda *et al.* 2006; Arvidson *et al.* 2011; Felitti *et al.* 1998; Harker 2018; Perry 2006; Siegel 2012). Early childhood trauma impacts the central nervous system, brain development and the overall health of the individual (Zeanah 2014).

Scholars have theorized and researched that the capacity to express full human potential is related to the brain's organization regarding perception of challenge in association with developmental experience (Perry 2006; Solomon and Siegel 2003). Abuse, trauma, neglect and other adversity can organize a developing brain to express a range of serious emotional and behavioral issues, along with cognitive deficits impacting growth and learning (Panksepp and Biven 2012; Van der Kolk 2014). Andersen and Teicher (2004) found that early exposure to stress and subsequent diagnosis in later childhood, adolescence, or adulthood with depression, substance abuse and post-traumatic stress disorder (PTSD) can be tied to sensitive periods of brain growth and maturation when specific regions of the brain are undergoing anatomical and functional development. This development is most susceptible to environmental influences and stress-related glucocorticoid hormones, as maladaptive exposure interrupts normative pruning with far fewer synaptic connections being made, particularly in the hippocampal region. These results support Carrion, Weems and Reiss's (2007) research findings that differences in hippocampal volume in children who are exposed to trauma and severe stress are more likely, due to the neurotoxicity of stress hormones such as glucocorticoids, to have resulting reduction within the hippocampus. This reduction increases cognitive issues such as memory or concentration, impairment with new learning and incongruence within the limbic system (Blumenfeld 2018; Carrion and Wong 2012).

Clinical implications for hippocampal and limbic system incongruence include the propensity for confusion with the past and present, memory impairment, flashbacks, nightmares and dissociative symptoms (Badenoch 2018). The corpus callosum is heavily myelinated, meaning the layers of lipid and protein substances around some axons greatly influence the velocity of impulse conduction among neurons (Moore, Dalley and Agur 2014) and this region is associated with hemispheric integration between the right and left hemispheres of the brain. High levels of stress hormones during infancy and early childhood are associated with suppressed glial cell division, a process which is critical for myelination to occur (Zeanah 2014). Research investigating the link between corpus callosum size and functioning for populations exposed to severe stress and trauma in early childhood demonstrated reduced corpus callosum size in children because of their history of maltreatment and PTSD (Carrion and Wong 2012; Keshavan *et al.* 2002). Disruptions in myelination and formation of the corpus callosum, due to exposure to severe stress and adverse experiences, yield high levels of hyperarousal and secreted stress hormones including cortisol and glucocorticoids during the first three to five years of life. These are moderately to strongly intercorrelated with sensorimotor function, visuospatial processing, executive functioning, language and general cognitive functioning impairment (Pears and Fisher 2005). Reductions in cortex volume have been found in prefrontal cortical white matter and right temporal lobe volume reduction in addition to reduction of volume within the corpus callosum (Harker 2018). Research is coalescing to demonstrate that child abuse and neglect create enduring psychological, behavioral, medical and social outcomes with long-term health consequences which increase morbidity and carry significant health care expense (Toth and Gravener 2012). The estimated annual cost of this issue, including both immediate needs of expenditures and the long-term secondary effects, are estimated at $103.8 billion (Wang and Holton 2007). Clearly, this is an issue which demands our attention to find early intervention solutions.

Propensity of misdiagnosis

We live within a world where diagnosis is necessary in the context of managed care reimbursement and is tied to considerable pharmaceutical interventions among providers. For example, the high prevalence of attention deficit hyperactivity disorder (ADHD) diagnosing includes a level of behavioral problems representing internalizing and externalizing behaviors. Many of the predominant symptoms classified by the American Psychiatric Association (APA 2013) include inattention/concentration symptomatology, in addition to hyperactivity or impulsivity symptoms, which can all be connected to trauma exposure. We can hypothesize that exposure to ACEs can lead to behavioral problems, including hyperarousal, that become confused with symptoms of ADHD. Hunt, Slack and Berger (2016) investigated this issue and describe a strong association within their data regarding early exposure to adverse experiences and ADHD diagnosis by age nine. This phenomenon is one experienced by Kelly, with subsequent treatment targeting an incorrect diagnosis. Considering the staggering cost of care for addressing childhood trauma and the propensity for misdiagnosis, we must not fail to address adversity within our assessment process. It is imperative that we have early intervention and assessment procedures with clinically appropriate, psychological and behavioral approaches facilitated by trained child providers who understand brain development, the impact of trauma on the nervous system and physiological functioning, while utilizing clinical applications which include the mind and body for healing ACEs.

Evidence-based practice

We often become trapped in an evidence-based world, meaning programs which have received acclaim and recognition as being evidence-based are often the manualized treatment protocols that offer an ability for randomized control trials. Transparency may be lacking within the methodology of the research and results are simply published as meeting significance. The treatment then becomes adopted by the public as reputable. These treatments can become accepted as guidelines for treatment with children; however, clinicians are failing to critically appraise the evidence and scope of the manualized treatment protocol or original intentions of the intervention based on population factors. We see agencies assign treatment protocols to clients as a "one-size-fits-all approach" for any diagnosis. The treatment may never have been researched to support the diagnosis it is assigned to. Sometimes research has inherent flaws within its design and data analysis, prompting the need for therapists and agencies to become better consumers of research products. A 2011 report from the Institute of Medicine (IOM) discussed in Whitaker and Cosgrove (2015) provides insight regarding the inherent problem:

> Most guidelines used today suffer from shortcomings in develop-
> ment. Dubious trust in guidelines is the result of many factors,
> including failure to represent a variety of disciplines in guideline
> development groups, lack of transparency in how recommendations
> are derived and rated and omission of a thorough external review
> process. (p.138)

However, the American Psychological Presidential Task Force (2006, p.273) stated: "Evidence-based practice in psychology (EBPP) is the integration of the best available research with clinical expertise in the context of patient characteristics, culture and preferences." They also state:

> There are many problem constellations, patient populations and
> clinical situations for which treatment evidence is sparse. In such
> instances, evidence-based practice consists of using clinical expertise
> in interpreting and applying the best available evidence while
> carefully monitoring patient progress and modifying treatment as
> appropriate... Research suggests that sensitivity and flexibility in
> the administration of therapeutic interventions produces better
> outcomes than rigid application of manuals or principles. (p.275)

There is a need for advocacy to allow behavioral health providers and child therapists to draw from the research literature while maintaining flexibility in selection of theory and its applications for client care. Rigid programs are not the solution. What Kelly experienced in her treatment history was assignment to a rigid behavioral-based protocol with limited flexibility. PCIT has efficacy for achieving results within Kelly's age group, but the manualized program was not designed for Kelly's presenting history, which resulted in an unsuccessful outcome.

A child in treatment can carry on average three to seven distinct co-occurring diagnoses found within the *Diagnostic and Statistical Manual of Mental Disorders* (DSM; APA 2013). However, through the lens of developmental psychopathology, almost all their presenting issues can be accounted for by the developmental injuries in the context of their caregiving system (Van der Kolk 2018). The guidelines that offer another approach to the creation of treatment planning move beyond a simple manualized program and encourage clinicians to think flexibly within their work and treatment planning.

Rather than simply labeling a client as "non-compliant" or failing treatment, the clinician can be encouraged to critically appraise their intervention plan and draw upon the power of a peer-reviewed process to find room for improving outcomes. The shortcomings of unsuccessful treatment are more aptly the responsibility of the clinician rather than the child within their care. Diagnostic assessment practices often fail to adequately assess for trauma and adverse experiences. We often fail to include environmental factors in formulating treatment assigned or taken on by therapists who, despite limited knowledge in child development, trauma or effective practices for treating developmental trauma responses, are expected by their agency to treat the client and work across the lifespan regardless of training or skill level.

The development of a safe, secure and therapeutic relationship in which there is trust and rapport is important for all therapies, but essential when working with children who have experienced relational trauma. Children with relational trauma often need opportunities to rework attachment difficulties. Bowlby (1969) described a process of revising internal working models to build a foundation of knowing security within relationship. Living in safe, predictable environments is essential for normative development and a requirement for our defense systems to "turn off" allowing us the ability to play, experience intimacy, collaborate with others and feel safe and loved (Briere and Scott 2006; Porges 2017). We are social beings; however, social engagement is not the same as social support and a central focus of treatment needs to include repair of the internal working model to help those traumatized find safety, security and meaning (Van der Kolk 2018). Repair in relationships may also best be achieved by those who have developmental trauma through learning resonance and synchrony from other mammals, such as dogs and horses, who can support the nervous system in a less threatening manner than a human could (Van der Kolk 2018).

Expressive therapies and movement

Expressive therapies and creative arts are responsive to the developmental and emotional needs of children, providing necessary experience to shape development. Axline (1969) demonstrated that play is the child's natural medium for self-expression. Children can express a wide range of emotions and cognitions through their play, and play is the most appropriate mode of processing experience for healing (Carey *et al.* 2015; Findling *et al.* 2006). Play provides balance and safety due to the symbolic nature of materials and child expression (Landreth 2001; Shelan and Stewart 2015); creative arts, including play and expressive practices, have a unique role in the reduction of trauma symptoms for those who have difficulty with verbal expression (Malchiodi 2008). Young trauma survivors with limited language, and those who are unable to put experiences into words, benefit from expressive arts because they offer a means of communicating ideas without words. Expressive therapies that include the integration of movement, art and music are vital components for the developing mind to formulate understanding of traumatic experiences (Gil 2006). Early intervention for children exposed to trauma and adversity through play therapy and expressive arts may shift the long-term health outcomes described by the ACE study.

Kelly's case demonstrated significant evidence of trauma exposure and adversity for early development. Kelly has been identified as neuro-atypical in development with sensory processing deficits and made gains through occupational therapy. Her symptoms and history were originally conceptualized by mental health clinicians as ADHD with separation anxiety, and a behavioral approach was prescribed as the evidence-based treatment intervention of choice with no documented communication or collaboration with occupational therapy. The top-down approach of mental health focused on extinguishing problem behaviors through various types of reinforcement to shift thinking and behavioral patterns, which simply did not work. Rather than revisiting the formulation of diagnosis and thinking about alternative treatment approaches, the child was blamed for the lack of process, with Kelly being labeled a failure and non-compliant with her treatment program.

Considering the overwhelming exposure to trauma between infancy and age six, we can better conceptualize Kelly's symptoms as those of exposure to violence and trauma, resulting in the re-organization of her brain as a brilliant adaptation to cope with her external environment. Based on her history and the knowledge of how adverse experiences impact brain growth and development, Kelly's case can be viewed through this lens and intervention can be approached bottom-up, with goals focused on lower brain integration for regulation. Porges (2015) provides a neurobiological model of understanding through the polyvagal theory. He describes the need for individuals to feel safe and physiologically calm. Van der Kolk (2018, p.31) furthers this idea:

> When our cries go unheard and our pleadings don't stop the abuse, this automatically releases the sympathetically based flight-fight system, or the parasympathetic unmyelinated immobilization shut-down response. It thus makes sense that children with trauma histories suffer from both externalizing and internalizing behaviors; they display both various degrees of unmanageable behaviors (these squeaky hells attract the most grease—and diagnoses such as ADHD and oppositional defiant disorder), and withdrawn self-isolation.

The adaptations of trauma to protect the self, identity, emotion, mind and physical body are often mislabeled as behavioral problems that need correction or extinguishment. However, what if these same behavioral problems were keeping the child alive within their environmental system? If we fail to understand the root etiology behind the behavior are we doing more harm than good?

Brain development

Discovering how the brain and nervous system works, in addition to the philosophical ideas behind the mind, have created an increase in interest and excitement from contemporary scientists. Understanding the diverse knowledge derived from the various levels of genetics, genomics, molecular and cellular biology, anatomy and system biology in addition to behavioral observation and psychology would be too vast an undertaking for any one body of work. Understanding the brain, body and mind will continue to be a lifelong journey of learning with contributions of research, education building and refining of our work.

The nervous system includes a network within the body that functions to manipulate and process both internal data and external information. The nervous system is specialized for rapid communication including nervous tissues, like all other organs, composed of cells creating networks, with the brain working as a central control station (Purves *et al.* 2012). There are estimated to be a hundred billion nerve cells (neurons) within the human brain and at least as many glial cells (Nolte 2009; Presti 2016; Siegel 2012) with an average of ten thousand connections directly linking among neurons, making the brain a highly complex yet organized structure (Applegate and Shapiro 2005; Badenoch 2008). These are the two basic categories of cell in a large and complex system. Neurons facilitate information processing and signaling (they are the lead actor within the production) while glial cells provide support (the supporting role to the neuron's lead role). The nervous system can be divided into two categories: peripheral nervous system and central nervous system (Nolte 2009). The peripheral nervous system includes pathways that move into all parts of the body and convey important messaging from the central nervous system (Moore *et al.* 2014). The central nervous system contains the brain and spinal cord, with the brain itself comprising many additional structures, all of which contribute to information processing of internal and external data entering the nervous system. The brain develops from the bottom up, with development of the neural tube moving forward to form the spinal cord and lower brain stem with further differentiation in the cerebellum and cerebral cortex (Nolte 2009). The brain continues this process of growth in a hierarchical manner with most of the brain organization occurring within the first four years of life (Perry 2006).

Epigenetic considerations

The field of epigenetics has provided us with an account for the effect that acute and chronic stress, particularly adverse childhood experiences, has on the brain and behavioral development of an individual (Lussier, Islam and Kobor 2018). Epigenetics, or heritable changes in gene expression, offers a way to deepen our understanding of illness etiology due to trauma exposure with transgenerational effects (Ramo-Fernandez *et al.* 2015). Epigenetics is defined by contemporary biologists as "how genetic material is activated or deactivated—that is expressed—in different contexts or situations" (Moore 2015, p.14). This is further explained by Moore as DNA operating not as an on/off light switch but rather like a dimmer switch; it can be turned on in small, moderate or large amounts or be fully "on" with any amount or variation in between. At the heart of stress response is the hypothalamic pituitary adrenal (HPA) axis connecting the central nervous system and endocrine system within our body. Studies investigating the changes in methylation within the HPA axis of lab rats have shown evidence of change due to maternal stressors impacting rat pup development, changing the gene expression within future generations of pups (Smart *et al.* 2015). Further research within genetic mice studies has tied chronic stress leaving "epigenetic markers," or changes that alter how DNA is expressed without altering its sequence, to health changes which parallel the long-term health effects of ACEs. This is evidenced through investigation of environmental influences on microRNA (miRNA) of sperm (Gapp *et al.* 2014; Hughes 2014). Gapp *et al.* (2014) report that injection of sperm RNAs from males exposed to trauma into fertilized wild-type oocytes reproduced the behavioral and metabolic alterations in offspring. Studies of chronic stress provide evidence that early exposure to stressful events releases peptides from the HPA axis, which has persisting influences on the brain and subsequent behavior (Sandman *et al.* 1997). Psychobiological stress occurring in pregnancy during fetal development yields disrupted emotional regulation, impaired cognition, decreased brain volume and associated learning and sensory system disruption (Sandman *et al.* 2012). This body of research supports the biological implications of adversity having multigenerational impacts through epigenetic factors.

Labonté *et al.* (2012) completed a study with human subjects, utilizing brain tissue from the Quebec Suicide Brain Bank of individuals who had abuse and trauma histories compared with brain tissue from non-abused individuals. The results of this study included a genome-wide methylation analysis, which supports research suggesting that early trauma and life adversity create a pattern of alternations for both hypermethylation and hypomethylation in several gene promoters. These gene promoters inversely correlate with gene expression throughout the whole genome. These findings are in accordance with studies of laboratory mice and rats (Labonte *et al.* 2012). Research within epigenetics demonstrates the phenomenon of child abuse and neglect creating enduring psychological, behavioral, medical and social outcomes with long-term health consequences that not only increase morbidity but shift genetic patterns for future generations (Harker 2018; Toth and Gravener 2012). Research shows that children and adolescents exposed to trauma have epigenetic influences on their HPA development and immune processes because their experience influences the next generation, with social and financial ramifications (Nugent, Goldberg and Uddin 2016).

Kelly's mother reported four out of ten adverse experiences within her own childhood; parental mental health illness, alcoholism in the family system, divorce and episodes of neglect. Chronic stressors during her own development, coupled with ongoing stressors of living within intimate partner violence, created the possibility of genetic alterations impacting sensory systems and mental health outcomes for Kelly. Considering the transgenerational impact of trauma, the overall estimate of financial cost to society for childhood trauma can be increased substantially as we project the cost of care for offspring of trauma survivors, which is why interdisciplinary work within the field of genetics is important for child mental health practitioners. Best practice treatment for child trauma must include research central to neurodevelopment and genetics as we navigate the implications of adverse childhood experiences.

Adverse experiences and the nervous systems

The central nervous system (CNS) consists of the brain and spinal cord and the peripheral nervous system (PNS) encompasses all additional parts of the body's neural networks (Presti 2016). This system (PNS) includes various sensory systems for the head (eyes, nose, ears, tongue) and the connections of these systems and the sensory data from the body's epidermis communicate with the brain. Systems which respond to touch, temperature and pain have receptors located within the muscles, tendons and joints which provide sensory information about muscle tension, body position and safety, allowing for control of movements within the neuromuscular system (Moore *et al.* 2014; Presti 2016; Sapolsky 1994). The nuances of life include our ability to register muscle tension, eye movements, tone of voice and cadence of speech in addition to our internal canvas of biological functions for heart rate, breath, blood sugar analysis, temperature—these are all woven within our body and brain and linked by the peripheral nervous system through the synchrony of the two branches of the autonomic nervous system (ANS): the sympathetic and parasympathetic (Van der Kolk 2014). The ANS regulates organs and internal functions including our heart rate, blood pressure, breathing and digestion (Presti 2016; Sapolsky 1994) with the relationship between breath and heart rate referred to as the respiratory sinus arrhythmia, an index of parasympathetic (vagal) tone to the heart

(Levine 2018). The sympathetic nervous system moves us forward like an accelerant while the parasympathetic provides slowing, acting as a brake to the process.

Table 2.1 Chart of sympathetic and parasympathetic nervous system

Sympathetic	Parasympathetic
Diverts blood flow to muscles	Diverts blood flow to core
Increases heart rate	Decreases heart rate
Originates in thoracic and lumbar regions of spinal cord	Originates in sacral region of spinal cord, medulla, cranial nerves 3, 7, 9, and 10
Activates fight-or-flight	Activates rest and digest
Utilizes chemicals such as adrenaline	Utilizes chemicals such as acetylcholine
Muscles constrict	Muscles relax
Stops bladder from eliminating	Stimulates your bladder to release
Increases airways and lung capacity; bronchial tubes dilate	Slows breathing; bronchial tubes constrict
Pupils dilate	Constricts pupils

The last component of the PNS is called the enteric nervous system, an intricate network of neurons creating connections within our gastrointestinal system; the enteric system has neural interconnections with the CNS and operates with impressive autonomy, regulating its own processes (Presti 2016). Therefore the ANS does not stand alone in a silo of biological operations but works in concert with the entire nervous system structures and brain including the amygdala, regions of the prefrontal cortex and the hypothalamus (Badenoch 2008). All structures play a role within the process we term "regulation," or the ability for the body to engage in a dance of synchrony moving toward balance within the nervous system, thus staying within the "window of tolerance" (Siegel 2012).

Connections between the CNS and PNS are through the spinal cord via one of twelve pairs of cranial nerves. The tenth cranial nerve became highlighted in work on the polyvagal theory (Porges 2017).

The theory assumes when the tenth cranial nerve, vagus and associated social engagement systems are in a state of optimal functioning, the autonomic nervous system can support health, growth and restoration (Porges 2017). Porges coined the term neuroception to describe our neurobiological systems as scanning the environment for safety, danger or threats to the nervous system. This could be in the form of physical danger, emotional danger or incongruence within the environment or interpersonal relationship. If we have achieved a neuroception of safety, the ventral vagus prevents the flight or fight response of our sympathetic nervous system and allows us to seek social engagement or to feel secure within our relationship or attachment system. The sympathetic nervous system will prepare us for danger within the system, aiding in our search for support; however, if help doesn't come or we experience a state of hopelessness and helplessness, the parasympathetic nervous system engages a dorsal vagal response to allow our body to slow. This is a strategy to conserve resources in the event death does not occur as we move toward collapse and dissociation. Experiences of perceived stress on the nervous system can be positive, tolerable or toxic. Positive stress has the potential of adaptive outcomes and is a necessary part of life for development. This type of stress helps us to obtain goals or create ambition toward new changes. Typically, this type of stress is short-lived and occurs within a relationship which is viewed by the individual as supportive. This permits for the opportunity of co-regulation, if needed, and supports a return to an internal state of calm where an individual or child can achieve mastery and empowerment. Tolerable stress is more challenging and longer in duration. If unrestrained, this type of stress can impact brain development and mental health functioning. Mitigation of tolerable stress can occur within caring relationships; however, tolerable stress can become toxic stress when it is prolonged. Toxic stress is the most severe and prolonged form of stress, occurring in confusing, disorganized attachment systems, with caregivers struggling to co-regulate heightened states of arousal or a lack of resources. Chronic neglect, abuse, exposure to violence, significant poverty and unsafe environments (home, neighborhood, war) all contribute to toxic forms of stress (Harder *et al.* 2012; Harker 2018).

Mind–body connection: impact of trauma and integrating movement through yoga

Post-traumatic stress disorder (PTSD) is now differentiated in the *Diagnostic and Statistical Manual of Mental Disorders (DSM5)* (APA 2013) for adults, adolescents and children, with criteria modified to guide clinicians towards diagnosis with children under six. PTSD follows exposure by directly experiencing or witnessing aversive or life-threatening events with the presence of intrusive thinking (children may engage in post-traumatic or repetitive play). There are often components of distressing dreams, dissociation and marked psychological and/or physiological distress. There is persistent avoidance of anything that may stimulate memory or association of the event and the individual may experience negative alterations to cognition and mood. PTSD is also associated with memory disruption, confusion or memory loss and individuals can feel awash with shame, guilt or blame regarding the event(s) perceived to be traumatic. PTSD shifts the nervous system with changes in arousal (hyperarousal or hypoarousal); dissociation may be a factor for those in hypoaroused states who have experienced trauma.

Classic PTSD is discussed in literature and research in differentiation to the theories underlying complex trauma or developmental trauma (Courtois and Ford 2013). Complex trauma is distinguished from a classic form of PTSD due to individuals having all the components of PTSD in addition to layered additional experiences of pain associated with relational/familial and interpersonal forms of traumatization (Courtois and Ford 2013). Exposure often includes chronic threats to the integrity of the self. Personal development is greatly impacted and the ability to interrelate with others becomes impaired (Courtois and Ford 2013; Malchiodi 2008). Freyd (1996) discussed this aspect of trauma through the lens of "betrayal trauma" in the context of a child experiencing sexual abuse, physical abuse or neglect from the person designated to care for and protect them. This complex trauma includes harm at the hands of the child's attachment figure, creating disorganization within the attachment and nervous system. The confusion resulting from betrayal trauma creates complexity that is not adequately addressed in our current diagnostic criteria for PTSD. A diagnosis of complex PTSD or developmental trauma is more appropriate to the type of adverse experiences and trauma children face. Complex forms of PTSD, which include disruption to attachment and the nervous system, benefit from a whole brain and body approach towards intervention. These interventions need to be enveloped within a safe and secure therapeutic relationship. Treatment centered entirely around cognitive processes or behavioral modification is often missing a large aspect of human experience. A missing component is the nuances and complexities of the nervous system as a result of the complex trauma in a child's neural development during prolonged and toxic stress states. Concurrently, most purist approaches to treatment can fail to include thoughts, ideas or narratives unique to the individual. Therapy facilitated from a holistic approach, drawing from research and practice-based wisdom, which integrates theory and incorporates the complexity of experience including body, brain and mind within social connections, creates the possibility for a deeper and longer lasting multi-generational impact for health.

The neurosequential model of therapeutics (NMT) is one way of providing a developmentally sensitive and neurobiologically informed practice for childhood trauma and adversity, in which clinicians can engage in problem solving and intervention (Gaskill and Perry 2014). The approach includes specific sequencing of experiences which are neurodevelopmentally appropriate and support the selection of specific therapies within a comprehensive therapeutic plan (Gaskill and Perry 2014). Often children who have experienced trauma and adversity enter treatment with the inability to regulate emotion and the physiological intensity of their feelings. Entering into a therapeutic space which promotes lower brain stem regulation and moves upwards into relational and emotional centers of the brain, ending in a cognitive engagement, yields successful results. We have found that offering the ability for lower brain stem activities (movement, breathwork, rhythm, music—humming or use of the "bee breath" in yoga, spinning and stretching) gives children the ability to prepare for more complex play or cognitive activities, whether they are child-led or therapist-directed depending upon the therapeutic process.

A moment to think...

Let's pause for a moment and begin with an activity. I (Michelle) was introduced to this activity through a seminar within my doctoral studies at the University of Pennsylvania. This simple activity has been helpful for clinicians thinking about the world of abused or traumatized children. This is best done if you can find a partner or possibly a trusted family member or friend who is brave enough to be your experimental test subject in this activity. Begin by orienting your partner to the activity by telling them they are about to take a timed number and word test. The goal is to record as many numbers as possible and answer the word questions when prompted in the time provided. When I'm in a large group, such as a classroom, and I say there will be a test describing that those who record the most numbers and answer the most questions correctly win...typically, those who have a naturally competitive temperament sit up straighter and ready their pencils with eager anticipation. As you read the numbers and questions, start out slowly on the list but increase your pace of reading as you go until you are reading through the numbers and questions at a brisk pace.

The activity looks like this:

8 97 5 45 98 2 72 845 974 1587 9 33 110

1865 2875 354 94 25 65 4564 87 7 1654 6876 6546

85 Name a Color 7894 65 45 5 8973 458 89 13 548 6541

8 3245 458 6 10 78 678 9874 6 9 41 23 87

Name a Genius 8787 45 6 98 456 265 421 86 487 65

47 5864 Name a Piece of Furniture 458 568 3 5698 12

45 4561 98 895 49 1245

Stop

Now ask your participant(s) the following questions:

1. What do you feel in your body? Sensations? Emotions? Describe the felt experience right now.

(Process this experience with your participant or group; look for commonalities in physiological sensations or cognitive processes.)

2. How many people chose the color blue? If not blue, was it red, green, yellow? A common primary color?

3. How many people wrote Einstein down?

4. Who wrote down a chair? If not a chair, was it a table, bed or other common piece of furniture?

This exercise is designed to highlight how, when our sympathetic nervous system becomes activated, we find ourselves with a more narrowed focus; this is because it is the same system that prepares us for survival. How can we possibly take the time to be creative when we're surviving? Could we have used our imagination and created new possibilities when we were feeling anxious or a threat? Did anyone select chartreuse or aquamarine for their color choice? Could anyone stop to imagine other inventors, physicists, mathematicians, artists or humanitarians that helped change the world through their genius? Did we choose a chaise longue or think of an antique grandfather's clock for our furniture choice? Nope. We typically get Einstein sitting on a blue chair for this activity. Why? Because it is very difficult to have a clear mind and think creatively if you are in a state of hyperarousal. Yet as expressive arts and play therapists we expect children to enter into a world of creativity and problem solve, create comprehensive trauma narratives and express their thoughts, sensations and emotions through the creative process. How can they possibly do this if they are flooded and in a state of hyperarousal?

The power of movement through yoga: bottom-up regulation

Yoga is not a new idea; it has been a part of human societies for thousands of years. The *ashtanga* (eight-limbed) yoga system of Patanjali provides one type of guidance or vision of yoga practice

(Sovik and Bhavanani 2016). Yoga is both a state of process and a goal; it is a *moksha shastra* (freedom teaching), a process leading to gradual freedom from various forms of human suffering (Sovik and Bhavanani 2016). Yoga offers an opportunity for the mind, body and spirit to yoke; the word yoga is a Sanskrit word, *yuj*, meaning to yoke or bind, and can be interpreted as a union of the mind and body. Philosophy of human suffering within yoga practice is rooted in the idea that suffering is a faction of the mind constantly caught in the past, projecting into the future, engulfed in worry about things that cannot be changed or may not happen and experiencing shame, guilt or blame towards the self for what is outside its power to change. Therefore, yoga philosophy centers human suffering around the notion that we remain stuck within our own cognitions and mind. This philosophy is also seen within acceptance and commitment therapy, or the ACT model (Hayes, Strosahl and Wilson 2016). The idea of accessing the full richness of our humanity includes experiencing unpleasant thoughts and feelings alongside the pleasant ones; ACT insinuates the need for movement to help free our minds from what feels trapped by incorporating the entire body and environment into human experience. Traditional talk-based interventions which draw heavily upon linguistics are analytical and predominantly center within the left hemisphere of the brain for reprocessing, as a result often falling short with clients continuing to experience the physiological and emotional impact of trauma. Connecting movement through yoga with psychological theories, facilitated by expressive arts, unites both hemispheres of the brain and body to fully support trauma recovery.

Most commonly, when we think of yoga we think of the poses and positioning of the human body in the variety of yoga postures to stretch and strengthen our frames. Poses include standing, sitting or lying down. Yoga poses have many physical and physiological benefits, from muscle toning to strengthening of joints, tendons and ligaments. Yoga has more recently been linked, in biomedical and psychophysiology clinical research trials, to providing support and benefit for the lymphatic and metabolic systems within the body (Khalsa *et al.* 2016). Yoga integrates *pranayama*, or the practice of mindful breathing, which calms and regulates the body. *Pranayama* promotes deep relaxation and meditation, incorporating mindfulness into the behavior of breath and reflection towards the self. The health benefits of yoga practice extend beyond strengthening the body and toning muscle, increasing physical strength to increase the stability of the entire physiology through stress reduction. All these aspects of yoga aid in regulation of the nervous system response. By decreasing the activity of the sympathetic nervous system, yoga can shift the hypothalamic pituitary adrenal (HPA) axis and reduce toxic stress, positively improving health outcomes (Khalsa *et al.* 2016).

The power of breath can be captured through this simple exercise:

Take a moment and breath rapidly for a series of breaths in short and shallow bursts.

Stop.

Now repeat this rapid shallow breath pattern.

Stop.

Begin breathing deeply. Slow inhalations, with your exhalations longer than your inhalations.

What did you feel inside your body? Did your heart rate accelerate slightly? Did you feel like you were becoming anxious or even experiencing a moment of panic? Did you become aware of a shift towards becoming slightly lightheaded, your thoughts maybe becoming less clear? What shifted with the slow inhalation accompanied by longer exhalations?

When we inhale we stimulate the sympathetic nervous system, and rapid breaths activate the system for a flight/fight response. If we sit with a client who is experiencing a panic episode or flooded in a state of fear, typically their breathing rate has altered to something similar to what you may have just experienced. If you experienced or observed someone else during the previous activity on how heightened states of arousal impact creative thinking, they were not necessarily able to think creatively or make connections. Exhalations, particularly slow exhalations with the release of the breath slightly longer than the inhale, stimulate the parasympathetic nervous system. This decreases our heart rate and brings us towards a more clear-headed state. Typically, our sympathetic and parasympathetic nervous systems work in synchrony, working together throughout the day to create a harmonious balance in the body. Inhalations and exhalations provide the heart with a steady, rhythmic state. A good heart rate is a measure of overall well-being (Van der Kolk 2014). This is important because, when we feel balanced, we can think more clearly and manage minor mood changes (frustration, sadness, disappointment, change in plans for the day). This creates flexibility and what we may consider to be even-temperedness. If you have experienced a high level of adversity in your life and are living in a state of chronic stress due to a trauma response, you're more regularly going to be off balance within your autonomic nervous system. Physical health will suffer, and you will encounter a greater number of illnesses, temper flares or tantrums, disrupted sleep cycles and a whole variety of mental health or physical ailments as a normative state. The core of yoga includes self-observation or the ability to become introspective (Gibbons 2015). Yoga provides consistency in practice for breathing and allows a child, possibly for the first time, to connect to their body in a way which provides feedback to understand their own nervous system, thus giving them the opportunity to build the skills needed for self-regulation, mastery and self-awareness. Many yoga programs include combinations of breath patterns (*pranayama*), poses or postures with stretching and meditation or mindfulness. The variation and intensity of these core components of yoga vary depending upon the school of yoga one is working from.

We often hear yoga and mindful meditation (*dhyana*) used conjointly or within the same context as mindfulness. Mindfulness creates the non-judgmental moment-to-moment awareness of our present experience. Mindfulness is often considered in professional literature as a form of experiential processing and a presence of mind, meaning attention, informed by our awareness of senses and observation to what is occurring in the present. This means we simply observe what is taking place, whether it is an external or internal experience (psychological, somatic, environmental) (Brown and Cordon 2009; Shapiro *et al.* 2011). This concept of mindfulness is compared to other forms of processing generally filtered through our cognitive appraisals, judgments, evaluations (of self, other or environment), memories, beliefs, ideals, morals or other cognitive manipulation (Brown and Cordon 2009). Mindfulness is often considered to be rooted in the fundamental capacity towards consciousness, particularly attention and meta-awareness (Brown and Cordon 2009). Typically, mindfulness is something we need to practice or train, in a sense, to strengthen and incorporate into daily living. Mindfulness is not simply a therapeutic practice, but a basic human capacity (Brown and Cordon 2009) The concept of stress reduction through mindfulness has become popular with the research behind mindfulness-based stress reduction (MBSR) created in 1979 at the University of Massachusetts Medical Center by Jon Kabat-Zinn and colleagues. MBSR was developed as an adjunct medical treatment combining ancient Buddhist practice and Western medicine (Kabat-Zinn 1993). It is an intervention that teaches us to attend to the present moment, in a non-judgmentally accepting manner, resulting in reduced symptoms of depression, anxiety or stress (Polusny *et al.* 2015). MBSR encourages the student to take a kinesthetic experience or object of focused attention (most commonly the breath) and when awareness strays from the object the student is encouraged to gently bring the focus of attention back into the mind, clearing all other thoughts or distractions (Brown and Cordon 2009). As we explore one school of thought within yoga practice in the next section, we will see that one of the eight limbs of yoga (*ashtanga*) focuses on the breath or *pranayama*, providing opportunity for enhancing mindfulness. This can create a connection for therapists who practice mindfulness or MBSR to integrate yoga into practice.

The practice of yoga can assist with a trauma response because those who have experienced trauma often are stuck in re-experiencing their past, which we in the professional circuit see as symptoms. Trauma survivors react through developing habitual behaviors or patterns of being, ways of thinking which may become rigid. This creates an inability to be flexible or make changes; emotions can become stuck in states of hyperarousal or hypoarousal or oscillate rapidly between the two states, resulting in rumination, avoidance, anger, distress, dissociation or collapse. Mindfulness through breath work has been shown to reduce pain and treat depression and anxiety, thereby reducing trauma symptomatology (Follette and Vijay 2009). Mindfulness encourages acceptance rather than avoidance and can facilitate both exposure to adverse emotions and offer opportunities to regulate within a secure and safe therapeutic relationship (Follette and Vijay 2009). Yoga in the context of therapy offers the ability to engage in mindfulness through *pranayama* and breath to support trauma symptom reduction. This creates an opening to think, concentrate or direct our attention, relax the mind and physiology and attend to the present without getting lost in the past.

The eight limbs of yoga

The eight limbs of yoga (*ashtanga*) provide discipline, guidance and vision for understanding yoga and its properties. The eight limbs are all important independently and support one another to work together towards a state of unity. The first two limbs are centered around self-regulation and begin with *yamas* (restraints) for controlling negative patterns or habits which may shift or diffuse energy within the individual. This focus allows for reflection of the individual's well-being (Sovik and Bhavanani 2016). Through identifying negative tendencies within cognition, which are disrupting health and wellness, we can begin to help those we work with foster positive cognitions to replace negative thinking patterns. The *niyamas* are positive habits which create patterns for living and guide our overall practice. This framework can also be seen within the work of Shapiro (2017) for trauma reprocessing utilizing eye movement desensitization and reprocessing (EMDR). Knowing where and how disciplines can connect or interact offer us the beginning for planning how to integrate the fields of study for intervention development.

Table 2.2 Limbs one and two of yoga practice

Yamas	Niyamas
Restraints and guidelines for interacting with the world (Social Ethics)	Positive habits, ways of interacting with the world to foster your own peace and harmony (Personal Practice)
Ahimsa: reverence, love, compassion for all things, kindness	*Saucha*: simplicity, purity
Satya: honesty, truthfulness and integrity	*Tapas*: zeal and sincerity, austerity
Aparigraha: awareness of abundance, fulfillment	*Swadyaya*: study and introspective analysis
Astheya: generosity, non-stealing	*Iswara Pranidhana*: wholeheartedness, vulnerability
Brahmacharya: balance, moderation of life's vital forces	*Santosha*: contentedness

The yoga poses include movements, ways of positioning the body, poses which by design are described with the foundation of bringing one comfort and joy. This is an important aspect of yoga to remember while working with those who have experienced human atrocity such as physical or sexual abuse and neglect. Finding comfort and joy within one's own body is not easy. The practice of teacher adjustments (which we may see in routine yoga classes at studios or health centers in which a yoga teacher helps move a participant into correct posture positioning) should not occur with this population. One of the fundamental purposes we're describing within this text is children finding peace, joy and comfort within their own body. Trauma disrupts the process of a child finding connection to the body because often in trauma what we see is a mind–body disconnect. This is a powerful protective mechanism to avoid pain, discomfort or reliving of the trauma experience. Allowing children the opportunity to feel what is comfortable to them is an important aspect of the work. To position their body in a "correct" form would be similar to us saying "you can't trust your own body to tell you what feels right or wrong." One aspect of incorporating play and yoga within this framework is to describe *asana* in more depth, creating awareness for the child in connecting to their body and being able to tell us when discomfort occurs. This assists the child in creating meaning behind their physiology, somatic processing and emotional experiences.

Table 2.3 Limb three of yoga practice

Asana
Movement, posture, poses (Comfort and Joy)
Comfortable positioning of the body, security
Mind–body connection
Connecting to the spirit
Experiencing stillness and infinity

Pranayama, or breath work, includes the time-honored yoga practice of honoring one's own breath. We can control, find mastery, through our own energy shifts by changes in breath patterns. Activating the sympathetic nervous system response or parasympathetic nervous system creates the ability for a child to find their inner "superpower" of managing and shifting their own rhythm to regulate physiology, mood and find a clear state of thinking.

Table 2.4 Limb four of yoga practice

Pranayama
(Mindful Breathing Practice)
Honoring the breath
Uncovering your own purpose
Light, enhancement of one's own energy
Life force, rhythm, patterns

Prathyahara is the beginning practice of meditation or training yourself to draw inward and begin deep introspective reflection. This includes understanding that we are taking in billions of bits of data through our sensory systems from the outside world. Shifting the focus away from outside distractions and moving that focus to what our inner experience is conveying is a fundamental aspect of yoga practice that we can tune out or miss, yet it allows us to gain a better perspective of the self and deepens our understanding of who we are in the physical space.

Table 2.5 Limb five of yoga practice

Prathyahara
Beginning the practice of meditation (Drawing inward/Turning inward)
Use of senses to understand the outside world are drawn close, turning away from stimulation and towards the self
Provides alternate inner point of attention (focus on the breath or energy)
Senses go inward
Contemplative reflection of our core

Dharana is a contemplative state, focusing concentration to a single point. This may be a single point of the self (breath, body part, heartbeat, etc.) or an outside stimulus (noise, light source, focal point) with the goal of reducing distractions of sensory data. Some may use a mantra or chant to help focus and this practice reminds us that the mind naturally wanders, and we simply need to pull that focus back to our focal object or chosen stimulus repeatedly. The length of time our awareness stays connected to the object or sensory experience of our choosing will move us into a space that is more prolonged and requires less effort to pull ourselves back into mindful focus. This brings us into a space of dhyana, or meditation, and a feeling of letting go.

Table 2.6 Limbs six and seven of yoga practice

Dharana	Dhyana
(Concentration, Contemplation)	(De-concentration)
Turning inward with focus	Dropping our efforts, letting go
Turning outward with focus	Meditation
Reduce distractions	

Stay present, connect to one thing	
Noticing when the mind wanders and bringing it back into focus	

The last limb of yoga practice is *samadhi*, or the state of union with the universe or world around us, finding tranquility and bliss. This is a process of feeling connected with ourselves, others and the outside world as we live in the present and our mind becomes free from worry and suffering.

Table 2.7 Limb eight of yoga practice

Samadhi
(Purity, Bliss, Tranquility)
Constant and complete harmony of the self with the world around us
Union of universal energy
Mindfully present
Freedom (mind becomes still from worry, suffering)

Yoga and play for therapeutic intervention

Combining yoga, play therapy and neuroscience philosophies can help bring a comprehensive treatment approach to children's mental health issues. Integrative approaches will involve utilizing multiple theories, aspects of theory and practice-based wisdom in specific timed sequences aimed at supporting the physical body, thinking, emotional state or psychosocial functioning. The goal is to help children heal by entering a relationship which can reorganize and make new connections through the type of inputs selected and by creating a secure base. Connection for children who have suffered adverse experiences relates to finding meaning and bringing their mind and body into a connected awareness. This releases them from a state of feeling trapped or stuck within a trauma response. The approach is a bottom-up method using breath, movement and rhythm to soothe distressed physiologies and calm the nervous system response to trauma. This creates the ability to find creativity and engage in problem solving (whether it is through directive or non-directive expressive arts approaches) while in a safe and therapeutic relationship. The therapist will also pay close attention to their own physiological process and cognitive state during a bottom-up approach, as this sensory data information about the child and therapy process is important for ongoing assessment and intervention. Therapists use the information within their own body to support children to become regulated and soothe distressed physiologies, as well as to connect with a child, conveying non-verbally the feeling of being seen and understood. However, clinical process work with colleagues is needed to ensure the therapist can maintain a state of well-being. This work requires the therapist to show vulnerability and openness and to enter a room with deep empathy and compassion. The cognitive processing or trauma narrative will occur when the other aspects (body, mind and relationship) are in harmony.

Autocatalytic model

How do we create change for children who have been impacted by trauma? What is the best theory to draw from for a treatment option? What are the evidence-based practices for this client? How do I intervene in session? What reflections should I make that best meet the needs of the child? How do I talk with parents to help them understand what is happening? What if I do something wrong and damage this child? Am I enough for this child?

These are all thoughts we have heard from child therapists engaging in treatment with abused and traumatized children. Depending on the level of adversity and complexity of the family system, such as high conflict divorce cases or domestic violence situations, the questions become layered with fear related to the court process or possibility of giving testimony. These questions, paired with research and clinical practice, prompted an opportunity to explore a new avenue for conceptualizing assessment, intervention and eventual graduation from care.

Sir William Osler, a renowned diagnostician and clinician, worked to teach medical students that "the good physician treats the disease; the great physician treats the patient who has the disease" (John 2013). This philosophy can be extended to mental health practitioners in that each client who comes to us represents a story; the story includes their presenting symptoms, problem they are facing, social situation, belief system and the larger ecological systems impacting their health and functioning. Only when we understand the entirety of the client can we begin to develop a plan for how to intervene in a way that creates lasting change.

We need to understand the story that shaped our clients, their past and present environment, the political or larger systems impacting health and have a strong understanding of how development occurs. The assessment process is critical and needs a deep appreciation of the child and family system. The assessment focuses on interrelated practices of biopsychosocial-cultural functioning across the life cycle through a person-in-environment process. Many clinics receiving referrals for abused and traumatized children have a policy and procedure that includes an intake specialist completing the assessment during a one–two-hour session prior to the assignment being made for a primary provider to continue care. We voice through this model that the assessment process must be completed by the trauma provider, because trauma treatment begins at assessment. This initial building of safety and rapport, thereby establishing routine within practice, needs to be completed by the trauma specialist. Assessment is also multi-faceted and must include a thorough review of all the systems impacting a child's life. The outcome of the assessment creates the beginning phase of selecting treatment approaches or interventions to serve as a catalyst for change within the child. Intervention and theory must be intentional and congruent for the therapist to be successful, creating change for the child that is long lasting or autocatalytic and self-sustaining.

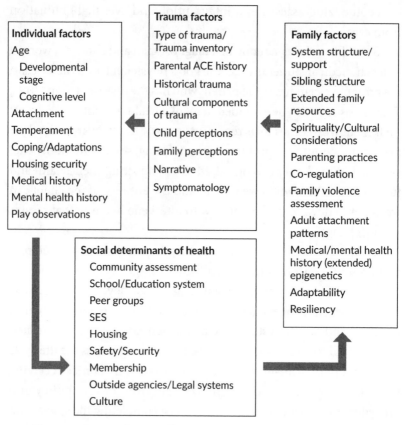

Figure 2.1 Autocatalytic quadripartite assessment (AQA) of child trauma

Repeatedly we'll hear therapists within treatment centers or programs discuss being forced into a treatment box. The program is solution-focused, provides only family strategic therapy or parent–child interaction therapy. The program has a policy or structure to adhere to an evidence-based practice model and therefore requires all therapists to utilize dialectical behavioral therapy for an intervention program. These are all examples of short-sighted system delivery models that fail to recognize that not every therapist finds congruence in a model, nor does evidence-based practice fit the complexity of the presenting issue. There is no one-size-fits-all approach to treatment and each child or family system is unique in the challenges they face. The background which brought them into the present-day space of our office will impact how we select our approach to intervene. A purist approach to treatment can miss valuable aspects of the child's worldview and ongoing needs throughout treatment.

An autocatalytic outcome results from a therapist having enough time for thorough assessment, flexibility and the ability to be innovative for theory selection, coupled with careful reassessment to determine results. Finding an autocatalytic outcome requires the ability to be prescriptive when necessary and can interconnect the right aspects of theory and intervention practice, creating a process which is supported by evidence, congruent for the therapist and best supports the client based on their assessment history. This includes the necessary knowledge of child development, biology and neurobiological considerations for trauma, regardless of theory or intervention style used.

Assessment must continue across the length of treatment combined with therapist self-care and accompanied by larger system support to ensure we are monitoring the effect of our input, as we are a catalyst driving the outcome. It is best practice to continuously assess if our therapeutic process is creating change through qualitative and quantitative measures and to receive feedback from various individuals within the client's ecosystem. It is also best practice to engage in peer review of the work, ensuring we have formulated our ideas about the case with outside evaluation. Additionally, a peer process supports the clinician in self-care through allowing room to discuss the impact of the case on clinician well-being. The correct selection of theories and modalities provides opportunity for integration to occur. The byproduct of this process becomes the catalyst through reorganization of the nervous system, and new neural networks are created which support integration of past trauma, allowing the client to maintain a balanced state without the intervention inputs from the therapist. The client becomes self-sustaining and is ready for graduation from care.

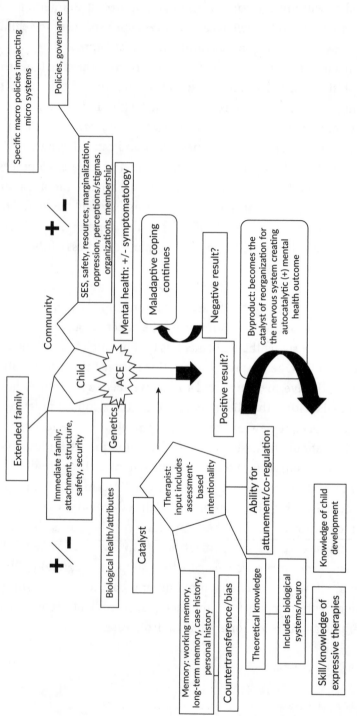

Figure 2.2 Autocatalytic model of practice

Thinking through an autocatalytic lens: the incorporation of animal assisted neurobiologically informed play therapy and yoga

Studies of the human animal bond discuss the emotional and physical health benefits of having an animal connection (Fine and Beck 2010). Children frequently seek comfort from their pets as a way to manage life stress, such as moving/relocation, starting school or family changes (Friedmann, Son and Tsai 2010; Katcher and Beck 2010) and animals are cited by professionals as enhancing socioemotional development (Fine and Beck 2010; Melson 1988). There is growing research discussing the implementation of animals within health care, citing that pediatric patients undergoing surgeries have experienced reduced stress when interacting with companion animals, as the animal moderates the stress response (Havener *et al.* 2001). Friedmann *et al.* (2010) discuss a series of studies in which blood pressure and heart rate were monitored while asking individuals to read aloud. This was compared to individuals asked to read aloud while in company with their own dog. The cases convey effects of lowered blood pressure and heart rate when the dog is present. However, in comparison studies with familiar and unfamiliar animals, the differences strongly suggest the attitude or attachment relationship with the animal is the key importance for stress reduction (Friedmann *et al.* 2010). A developed relationship with an animal in the life of a child exposed to adverse experiences may be a factor in mitigating the stress response of adversity, thus serving as a protective resource.

One area of our trauma practice includes a specialized form of play therapy integrating animal assisted human health, play therapy, neurobiology, movement and attachment theories. Animal assisted therapy (AAT) has built upon the benefits of the human–animal bond to assist the therapeutic process. AAT is defined by the Delta Society and discussed by Kruger and Serpell (2010) as:

> a goal directed intervention in which an animal meeting specific criterion is an integral part of the treatment process. AAT is delivered and/or directed by a health service provider working within the scope of their profession. AAT is designed to promote improvement

in human physical, social, emotional and/or cognitive functioning. Key features include: specific goals and objectives for each individual and measured progress. (p.34)

Animal assisted interventions (AAI) are defined as "any intervention that intentionally includes or incorporates animals as part of a therapeutic or ameliorative process or milieu" (Kruger and Serpell 2010, p.36). We emphasize the need for handlers to achieve credentialing and meet specific criteria standards for incorporating animal assisted human health therapies and interventions into their practice. VanFleet and Faa-Thompson (2017) discuss that when utilizing animal assisted play therapy in practice, advanced training in both animal assisted human health and play therapy is required. We agree with this and embrace Butler's (2013) advocacy for building upon foundational knowledge while expanding theory or practice; not clinging to established practices rigidly but being progressive and embracing new concepts grounded within past frameworks. We found the traditional approach of animal assisted play therapy could be expanded upon, built upon and enhanced for innovative trauma work including movement. This prompted us to begin researching and studying through single case design how to incorporate neurobiology and our conceptual knowledge of physiology into the work. We created an animal assisted play therapy program, building upon the work of researchers in both animal assisted human health and Van Fleet's work of play therapy, to combine play therapy and AAIs with neurobiology and movement. At the institute, we want to ensure best clinical practice with the populations we serve. Relying on the same selection tools as other certification programs for AAT and using all the same criteria or role expectations for dogs within play therapy needed more development for enhancing trauma interventions. To ensure our working dogs were well cared for in a therapeutic setting, which had complex and often stressful factors of trauma reprocessing, we needed to research and refine the approach to align with trauma work. We considered it our obligation to become advocates for balanced therapeutic and educational interventions in which the dogs were specifically selected for trauma support (Butler 2013). Therefore we developed this innovative program to engage our therapy dogs in animal assisted play therapy, blending neuroscience and movement into the process for enhancing regulation and trauma recovery which we termed "animal assisted neurobiologically informed play therapy." Canines within our institute have achieved certification in this model or are working towards that certification under supervision with their handlers. We define animal assisted neurobiologically informed play therapy (AANPT) as:

> A way of being in a harmonious relationship with both a child client and animal partner. AANPT utilizes interpersonal neurobiology to create a triangle in which an animal meeting specific criteria becomes an integral part of the treatment process. Animals join trained and certified play therapists in providing children a safe and nurturing space for empathy building, reduction of stress, emotional regulation, engagement in theory of mind and to help children build mastery for overall symptom reduction. AANPT provides children with the opportunity to integrate the negative effects of perceived challenges or adverse experiences, thus reestablishing a sense of power and control within their lives.

The features of AANPT include the concept of the animal becoming an integral part of treatment through the natural tendency the canine has of attuning to emotions. Therefore the animal mirrors the child's emotional state and nervous system response. This is observed through the lens of self-psychology, as Heinz Kohut defined in his theory construct regarding the "self-object experience" (Flanagan 2016a). The self-object experience occurs in development through formation, cohesion and achievement of a balanced sense of self through relationship with others (objects) incorporating principles of interpersonal experiences or "self-object experiences." Kohut describes the self-object experience as feeling recognized and affirmed, accepted by another, being able to assert oneself against an available and responsive other, feeling able to elicit a response from the other and having the other attuned to one's shifting moods and emotions, thereby co-regulating the process within the self-object experience (Melson 2001). This is a concept of AANPT and integrates the theory within the therapeutic process.

The principles of interpersonal neurobiology and attachment align with much of this theoretical framework and are components of the process behind AANPT. The most devastating effects of trauma occur within the primary attachment relationship, contributing to a developmental trauma response. Grounding within neuroscience of a secure attachment relationship allows for the opportunity to move toward a deeper approach to the work including the central importance of interpersonal experiences. This provides external variables to modify the synaptic connections, thereby enabling an individual to achieve new levels of flexibility, trauma symptom reduction and balanced forms of self-regulation (Siegel 2003). Stern's (1985) work with infant development informs and describes the central ways the self develops within interpersonal relationships during the critical early years of development. Daniel Stern articulated: "Without the nonverbal it would be hard to achieve the empathic, participatory, and resonating aspects of intersubjectivity. One would only be left with a kind of pared down, neutral 'understanding' of the other's subjective experience" (2005, p.80). We often rely too heavily on language and talk interventions; this research gives rise to the use of animals in expressive arts practice. The need for interpersonal relationships through modern attachment theory (also known as regulation theory) is a foundational lens to AANPT. Consistency, safety, routine and authenticity are requirements for the mind and body to find congruence within the environment and achieve a stress-reduced state within their window of tolerance (Schore and Schore 2008).

Dogs are inherently well suited for forming authentic relationships and integrate well into the play therapy setting. Children describe animals in this process as a reassuring presence during times of worry or fear, as they offer protection and help with loneliness. The dogs listen intently to their stories, provide support and give them an unconditional feeling of being wanted or loved. Jane Goodall and Marc Bekoff (2002) describe in their book *The Ten Trusts* that many animals show emotions that are similar if not identical to what we call fear, joy, anxiety, jealousy, love, sadness, compassion, anger and grief, and it is the shared emotions, the expression and similarity of these and their physiological and anatomical basis, which links animals to us. Dogs bring authentic presence and empathic understanding, often serving as a conduit for regulation with children. Dogs are playful and tap into the child's natural language for play. They interact in a way that is non-judgmental and accepting, truly embodying a client-centered approach infused with empathy. Dogs connect with others and mirror the emotion within the room, experiencing the physiological impact of trauma as any therapist would who is attuned within the process. Therefore, it is necessary the dog has opportunity for its own regulation and a handler who understands the importance of working with animal behavior, rather than issuing commands of correction to curb animal behavior.

Principles of movement through yoga offer opportunity for the child and animal alike to utilize the space and follow their body's natural cues to achieve a state of equilibrium. Multi-sensory experiences, including touch by petting or sinking fingers into the deep fur of a dog creates a kinesthetic regulatory opportunity, accessing the lower brain stem for bottom-up intervention. This allows associations to be made by children, assisted by the therapist, to move back into a window of tolerance and out of a state of hyperarousal or hypoarousal, thus building mastery. The feel of a dog's heartbeat is another cue utilized by children. A dog's resting heart rate is 60–120 beats per minute in small dogs and 60–100 beats per minute in large dogs (Aiello 2016; Klein 2013). This is in close parallel to a human's resting heart rate of 60–100 beats per minute (Moore *et al.* 2014). We can utilize a stethoscope in play therapy practice and we often utilize pulse oximeters; both can be purchased at low cost for therapists. A pulse oximeter will provide a digital readout to a child of their heart rate when gently clamped on their finger. Use of a stethoscope will allow a concrete prop-based representation of the heart rate for the dog, in addition to the child resting their hand on the dog's body. The dog naturally moves within a model that allows for free expression and can be tied creatively into yoga practice. Yoga poses which foster a parasympathetic response include breath work utilizing *pranayama* to engage the process and bring the nervous system back to a regulated state. This is one example of how psychoeducation about the sympathetic and parasympathetic nervous system can be incorporated through AANPT into practice with concrete prop-based education in real time.

Training and handler knowledge of AANPT involves in-depth knowledge of animal behavior as well as a securely attached relationship between the canine and handler. Trust and familiarity are essential between animal and handler as the natural activation the dog may experience during a session will be monitored and co-regulated during the process by the handler or therapist. It is unrealistic to assume a dog will not experience states of distress if you are engaging a child in trauma treatment. The child will experience distress at times as they reprocess adverse events. When a therapist allows a dog to be authentic they will mirror the child's emotional and behavioral system in session. Trained therapists in this paradigm utilize the opportunity to model adaptive coping through breath work and other forms of movement to include yoga. They may engage in cognitive reframes and bring the child (and animal) back into a state of equilibrium.

When the nervous system of a dog is activated they often naturally engage in a "bow" or "downward dog pose." Dogs have other stress signals including head-turning, blinking or squinting, licking lips, drooling excessively, yawning, shaking or moving in circles and/or pacing (Butler 2013). Children begin to recognize the behavior and therapists can choose how to reflect the dog's behavior back to the child. This is demonstrated within Kelly's case. Upon assessment it was discovered that Kelly had both a need for movement and a significant fondness for dogs. This created an opportunity to link, using the framework from an autocatalytic model, directive and non-directive AAIs, interpersonal neurobiology, play therapy through a trauma-focused lens and yoga into her treatment planning for reprocessing adverse experiences. During a particularly intense session with Kelly, in which a bear was hiding "somewhere" in the room (which we couldn't see, but we could hear), she commented about Apollo's (a golden retriever therapy dog) pacing and panting. She wondered aloud:

Kelly: Why does he do that?

Michelle: (choosing to reflect through physiology with the intention of orienting Kelly back to her own body) Hmmm... well, I feel like my stomach is tied up in a knot, there is a bear somewhere in our room that I can hear but cannot see and I feel like I can't breathe because of worries...maybe Apollo is feeling that worry too, knowing there is something out there that could be scary. He's trying to take care of his body so that he can think more clearly and stay safe.

Kelly: I feel like I have ants in my pants! My belly hurts too, and I feel a little sick. (large arm movements and big full body gestures)

Michelle: (taking a full yoga breath with controlled arm movements)

Kelly: (takes a big breath mirroring the arm movements)

Apollo: (moves into downward dog)

Kelly: (giggles, moves into downward dog)

Kelly and Apollo look at each other and Apollo gets out of position, walking over to lay on the floor up against Kelly. Kelly lies down and places her head on his side. I sit next to Apollo gently massaging his body where I know he likes to be rubbed along his shoulders at the base of his neck. I breathe long and slow breaths. He visibly calms and rests in a relaxed manner.

Kelly: It's OK boy, it's OK boy...I know the bear is scary. We're safe together.

Michelle: The bear was scary. We're taking care of our body and are safe now together.

Kelly: Hey, I can hear Apollo's heart!

Michelle: Really? I wonder what your heart is doing?

Kelly: (gets up and goes to the medical play toys and picks up the pulse oximeter, placing it on her finger) What does it say?

Michelle: It says 121.

Kelly: That's bad.

Michelle: That doesn't sound good to you.

Kelly: It's because of the bear. The bear makes our hearts bad.

Michelle: Not knowing where the bear is or if he may hurt us makes me feel scared and then my heart becomes fast too. I wonder if it is my body trying to help me and my body is giving me this clue that there is danger and I needed to find a way to feel safe. I'm just going to take a big breath. (takes a full yoga breath with accompanying arm movements and then another, narrating the feel of the breath)

Kelly: (watching) We can be safe together and Apollo is a good guard dog, he will bark if a bear comes again. We should make a potion while he keeps guard that keeps bears away.

Michelle: It sounds like we have an idea and a plan. Looks like thinking is clearer when our hearts don't feel bad. I like the way I feel after two deep breaths.

Kelly: Apollo is smiling!

Michelle: Maybe he likes your plan too!

Kelly: (visibly breathes in deeply) He does like this plan. Apollo! You are on guard dog duty. (walks over to Apollo with her stethoscope) I think his heart isn't fast.

Michelle: (noting the continued relaxed posture of the dog, no stress signals apparent) Yup, he looks ready for you to make that potion.

AANPT assumes that if you are bringing a dog into treatment you are doing so within best practice to maintain ethics and welfare for both the child and animal partner within interaction. Safety considerations for both child and dog are seriously evaluated during the initial assessment period. The therapist is consistently monitoring their own physiology as the dog will look to their handler for guidance and reassurance. The therapist is monitoring the child's physiology, emotion and behavior as their nervous system will be registered within the physical space by handler and dog. The therapist is also monitoring the animal's physiology and noting stress cues or distress signals. The process of co-regulating the child and dog through modeling and direct intervention is critical for ensuring safety and ethics are maintained in the process. We want to skirt the edges of the window of tolerance, not flood the child during trauma work. We also want to maintain our canine partner's window of tolerance during AANPT. There will always be clients who are not best suited for AANPT. The therapist will need to make decisions about the integration of this model during treatment.

Neurobiology, epigenetics and child development are fascinating subjects that will continue to be cultivated as our field advances in medical technology for understanding mental health phenomena. The importance of careful evaluation of research and what is advocated for as evidence-based practice will continue to require scrutiny from the professional clinician. Utilizing historical knowledge alongside current science while applying critical thought and practice-based wisdom can create movement for therapists to discover how to refine, build upon or develop new ways of intervening for trauma. There are many possibilities for creating new approaches for child trauma treatment by thinking expansively, outside the box, connecting the wisdom of interdisciplinary fields.

CHAPTER 3

Non-Directive and Directive Yoga and Play Therapy Practice

CASE EXAMPLES: KELLY, ANNA AND EMILY

Kelly

Kelly's first session began with a child standing in the center of a playroom staring at many toys representing significant options for play. It is not uncommon for children to enter a play space for the first time and experience emotional overwhelm. Kelly's father accompanied her to this first session, and she held his hand but just stared at the floor. Kelly's father worked in construction and owned his own business. I knew from a phone call the previous week that bringing Kelly to this session had been important to him. Kelly's school had been insistent upon therapy to stop the occurrences of fecal smearing. I stated, "sometimes there are almost too many choices when you enter a room like this for the first time." Kelly looked up as I knelt to become smaller, to meet her at her level. I explained the play therapy room was a space where she got to be herself and choose, it was a space where she could be anything she wanted to be or do what she needed to do. I told her that I might have questions from time to time, but she got to choose how to answer and that some children preferred to show me using the toys rather than talking with words. The most important thing was to remember this was a room where we were both to feel safe and that she would decide how to spend her time. This is a common opening I utilize to orient children to the play therapy space. My intention is to set the tone of safety and choice, creating a client-centered strengths-based experience. Kelly's father interjected at that moment.

> Dad: That's nice, but Kelly can talk. She is here to work on things, not play with toys and waste time.

> Michelle: Playing with toys can be a gateway into understanding problems. The toys can become the tools we need to build a story or explanation for what is happening. The toys help us make something abstract like anxiety or worry into something concrete which helps us think through issues. This is something like a house drawing versus let's say, building the actual physical house structure.

> Dad: Well, I don't want her to just play with toys and you watch.

> Michelle: Fair enough, why don't we build something together today using the toys?

> Kelly: (speaking for the first time and looking up with a worried expression) That would be OK, right dad?

Kelly's father agreed to this and they both followed me over to the sofa and coffee table. I pulled out a large piece of paper to create a family play genogram.

We feel that one of our primary jobs as child play therapists is to put family member concerns at ease and find new ways of connecting, even with the most skeptical critics who walk through the door. This may be a sibling or a parent who enters a session and needs concrete explanations, psychoeducation or reassurance about the process. Family sessions have an inherent need for structure; either we don't want a parent to become overwhelmed with emotion or we need to structure the session by providing coaching or skill building. This occurs with preparation during a parent consultation, and modeling during family sessions, to ease them into the process. We find family sessions often require structure when multiple members enter into the process. A therapist will need a plan for the session, organizing the time, especially if multiple children are involved. Chaos can quickly emerge in these situations if one is unprepared to facilitate multiple members working together.

Family play genograms

The family play genogram is a tool introduced by Eliana Gil (2015) which provides an excellent framework for capturing family systems through playful intervention. This tool builds upon McGoldrick, Gerson and Petry's (2008) work incorporating genograms within assessment and intervention. This family therapy task asks family members to select a miniature that best represents thoughts and feelings about everyone in the family including the child (Gil 2015). This allows for a process to unfold which incorporates the usefulness of putting what is often a complicated web of family connections into a concrete representational form for children to see, touch and contribute to in ways that are meaningful, as it utilizes their natural method of communication: play.

Kelly and her father sat down at my coffee table and began the process of creating a family map (genogram) with my help. I find with young children the form or specific nature of the genogram construction is less important than the process, therefore becoming less rigid about the technical nature of correct genogram construction can be helpful. The most important aspect is utilizing a key to track patterns. I will have children use all sorts of shapes and lines as they become active in the creation and simply keep track on the side of the genogram paper what they meant by the shape or line designation. Kelly used triangles to represent women within her family and squares for men. She used hearts for children and added paw prints for the animals in the family. Kelly's father took an educator role during this process, providing instruction and correction as they worked together to create the map. Kelly looked at him often and asked if she "got it right" frequently. Once we were all in agreement that the family members who needed to be on the map were placed on the map, I added the prompt for creating a family play genogram.

Michelle: Alright, now why don't we go on a scavenger hunt of sorts around this office. There are many, many toys, big and small, art supplies and other odds and ends you can choose from to represent your thoughts and feelings for each person in the family.

Dad: Yeah, you've got a lot of crap in here.

Michelle: (choosing to roll with the resistance) I do! We can use the whole office to find an object that represents our thoughts and feelings about who each person is, everyone in your family, not forgetting yourself. Once you find the object or several objects representing yourself and your family members, bring the items back to the map and we'll put it right on our drawing.

Kelly: Do you want to pick out the toys, Dad?

Michelle: You both get to pick out toys in here. Your Dad can choose, and you can choose because you will have different thoughts and feelings about each member of the family. Are you ready, Dad?

Dad: I guess. Let's get this done.

They moved around the room selecting objects. I enjoy opening the family play genogram up to the entire space rather than just a focus on the sandtray miniatures, as I've had insightful objects come back to represent family members over the years. I've had children select objects like the bottle of glue from the art supplies shelf to represent a mother who is interpreted as "holding the family together" during times of adversity and struggle. I've also seen objects like my *Perplexus* represent the entire family at the end, with a child saying, "My family is like this maze, you never know what is going to happen." Kelly and her father selected handfuls of miniatures and other objects. Returning to the coffee table, they began placing their objects on the map.

Dad: Why is that on my name? (looks pointedly at Kelly)

Kelly: (picks up a what had been a comic book villain character and hurriedly goes back to the shelf; she returns with a baker) I meant to get this one and made a mistake. This is for my Dad because he cooks me dinner and takes care of me.

Michelle: You decided to go to the shelf and get this man who looks like he is mixing a bowl and getting ready to make dinner.

Kelly: (pointing at a penguin) This is my Mom, she is a penguin. This is me, I am this girl (pointing to a plain *Playmobil* child character).

Michelle: What feels important to you about this girl?

Kelly: She is small.

Dad: I chose this beautiful princess to be you (places it on the map).

Kelly: (picks up the small child and removes her) OK.

Dad: You can keep both. Here is what I chose for me and your Mom (he places a man holding a bow and arrow for himself and a paint brush for Kelly's Mom). I'm this hunter because I like to bow hunt, and this is your Mom because she paints.

Michelle: Does this look complete to you or are we missing anything?

Dad: This looks good.

Michelle: What do you think, Kelly?

Kelly: This is fine.

Michelle: Alright, why don't we have a look around the room so that you know what kinds of things are here when you come back.

Kelly: OK.

Kelly explored the space for the last few minutes of her session, asking questions about items that were unfamiliar to her and if other kids came to play in the room. My goal was to give her the opportunity for movement and normalize the experience of how the room could be a space for children and families to talk or play. Kelly and her father left the office together and walked down the hall. The entire experience was layered in sadness and seemed to hold a buzzing intensity.

Kelly arrived the following week with her father. I greeted them in the waiting room and, as he began to stand up, I asked if Kelly felt like coming back to play on her own that day. She nodded her head as her father began to protest. I kindly reminded him of the different kinds of appointments, individual, family and parent-only appointments and that having time with just Kelly was important. He reluctantly sat back down. Kelly audibly breathed in the hall and smiled at me. Kelly asked, "What are we going to do today?" I responded, "We can decide to do whatever we need to do. I'm curious what we'll choose."

Kelly walked into the playroom and stood in the middle of the room looking around. She finally said, "I don't know what to do." I stood next to her looking around the room feeling nervous, therefore simply said, "I feel a little nervous when there are this many choices and I don't want to make a mistake." Kelly breathed out with a long exhale: "Me too." Sometimes launching right into non-directive play therapy can feel overwhelming for children. I chose to direct the session, beginning similarly to where we ended last time, with the aim at creating a window of opportunity for her to begin directing her own work.

> Michelle: Do you remember last time we met and you asked me about other children coming to the playroom?
>
> Kelly: Yes, you said other children came here too!
>
> Michelle: I did, and they do. One of the things we didn't talk about was yoga and dogs.
>
> Kelly: (giggling) What?
>
> Michelle: Right? Sounds silly.

My goal was to begin the dance of trust. I knew Kelly needed time to orient to the process, determine if I was consistent and see if I was congruent with affect and communication. I wanted to give her information and break the ice with a little humor. I began to tell her about Apollo the golden retriever therapy dog who often worked with me. She (possibly for the first time) truly looked engaged and had a spark of happiness. I brought down off the shelf a stuffed animal wearing a miniature version of Apollo's vest along with a picture of Apollo and talked with her about his role and how we could all play together, if she would like him to join us. She agreed and immediately asked for him to come in and play. I told her I would bring him next time and then we could have proper introductions. She agreed, saying "We have a deal, right?" I told her we had a deal and that I wouldn't forget. I brought my planner down from my desk and wrote on the following week it was an "Apollo day." Kelly nodded her head and said "Good."

I then introduced her to the idea of movement through yoga, beginning with asking her if she knew about yoga or had ever participated in yoga before. Kelly told me she knew what yoga was because she had seen her Mom doing yoga at home. I told her that we could decide when and how we did yoga during our time together and brought her a stack of cards with yoga poses, including modified poses children had created to help with storytelling. I introduce yoga in this way to explain that it could be helpful in telling a story with your whole body. We could use the mats like a stage (I pointed to a corner where rolled mats were stored) by moving our bodies to tell the part of the story we needed to anytime we wanted. I explained to Kelly, in my introduction to yoga, that it is also a way of helping our bodies when we have big feelings. We could take a big yoga breath or move as we needed using the poses as we wanted or moving our bodies like a dance. I asked if she would like to pick a card and we could both try the pose. Kelly looked through the stack and giggled, "I think I found Apollo's favorite pose." I looked at the card with the classic "downward dog" pose. I laughed and told her she was correct, and I got on all fours to do my best downward dog, adding a bark and a tail wag. She squealed and did the same barking and laughing. I asked her if she had any questions and instead she asked me, "Can we play the family game with these cards?" Not wanting to pretend I knew something I didn't, I answered with confusion, "I'm not sure I understand, but I want to play the family game. Can you tell me more?" She looked at me, "You know like last week." Clarity struck me then, and I smiled, "Oh, I understand! Thanks for explaining to me and of course we can play. Would you like to explain to me how it works?" This is how I stumbled across a family yoga genogram.

Kelly explained we were going to get out the family map and she would pick the yoga card that went with the family member. We were both to act out "playing yoga" with the pose. The only input I added was the opportunity for Kelly to "choose a pose" of anything she could think of if a card wasn't there when she needed it. Or she could choose a miniature or toy and we could decide what the yoga pose might look like to help with our storytelling. Kelly, truly animated now, said, "Yes!" jumping up and down. Kelly rolled out her family genogram from last week's session. She remembered exactly where I said I stored all the art and activities kids decided to leave in the playroom for me to keep safe. She seemed to know where every item was stored as she moved around the room "preparing" for the yoga family map activity she had created. She picked up a miniature here and there, "This doesn't go here, it was over there last time," placing it back where it belonged. She was right, of course. A child's sense of order is powerful, especially for a child who has experienced adversity and trauma. She mapped the room last session and needed to "right" her space before beginning the play.

> Kelly: (pointing to her mother on the map and stating with conviction) She's a penguin.
>
> Michelle: I remember she was a penguin last week. That feels important to me.
>
> Kelly: It is important. Penguins love their babies.
>
> Michelle: Well that is important indeed.
>
> Kelly: (pointing at a yoga card which displayed "frog pose") This is a penguin pose.

Michelle: (getting in "penguin pose") I'm in penguin pose.

Kelly: (moving into "penguin pose" as well) Me too. This is me (shows me "child's pose" and moves into position).

Michelle: (moves into child's pose) I wonder what the penguin feels thinking about her child?

Kelly: She's scared for her and wishes her baby was safe (getting up). This is a dad's pose (points to a card which showed "cobra pose").

Michelle: (moving into cobra pose) I'm in cobra pose, is this the right one?

Kelly: No, this is a dragon pose (moves into cobra or "dragon" pose).

Michelle: Now I'm wondering what the dragon would say.

Kelly: (hissing) You are a stupid girl, get over here.

Michelle: I don't think I want to go over there.

Kelly: You wouldn't. That's how you get dragon breath.

Michelle: That doesn't sound good at all.

Kelly: It's not (gets up and walks to the miniatures, selecting a bear). This one is my grandfather. He was eaten by a bear.

Michelle: He died because of a bear.

Kelly: Yes, and he is a bear now. This is bear pose (moves into cat pose). HE ROARS!

Michelle: (roaring too)

Kelly: Bears could fight a dragon I think.

Michelle: I wonder if that would make us safe?

Kelly: (gets back into child's pose) It's better to be small.

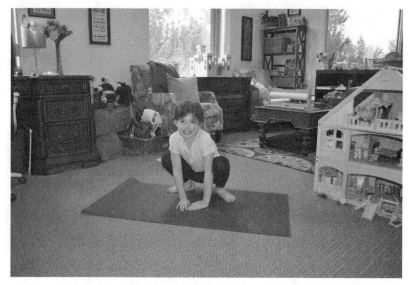

Figure 3.1 Example: "Penguin" pose

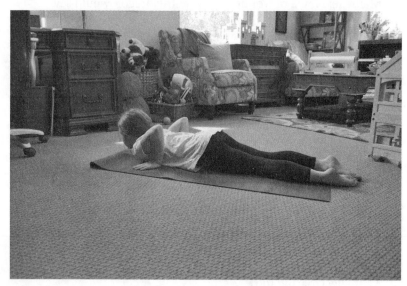

Figure 3.2 Example: "Dragon" pose

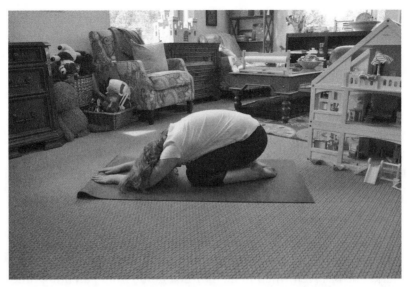

Figure 3.3 Example: "Becoming small" in child's pose

Kelly got up from the pose and moved into other play behavior, shifting the session away from the family yoga genogram and toward other aspects of her life or identity. She shifted through the session neurosequentially, starting with movement into relational work and ending with cognitive processing. She stated toward the end of session, "I like coming here. I like being here." I looked at her and said, "I'm glad you're here and I get to be here with you." As we left to return to her father she asked more than once when her next appointment was. This became a routine aspect of ending her session, asking about her next appointment as we moved down the hall. We entered into the waiting room and we said our goodbyes. The reassurance was important for her, knowing that she had a time and space in therapy the following week.

Kelly's case continued to progress, with a child whom I suspected had more going on within the family system than had originally been discussed during intake or was available within her medical history. It is important to remember we're not forensic interviewers, our role is to provide a safe therapeutic space for children to engage in clinical psychotherapy. To be both a forensic interviewer and a child therapist entails us engaging in two roles. This becomes problematic for any case, especially those which involve prosecution. This was an important distinction to explain to Kelly's mom during scheduled parent consultations. Kelly's mom was scared for her daughter and became tearful during those initial meetings. "I know something is going on, but I don't know what it is. I feel so helpless." I reminded her that if she suspected any abuse, or had concerns, the best course of action was to schedule an appointment with the pediatrician for a medical review and they could determine if a referral to our pediatric forensic interviewing team would be appropriate. She could also call the local Department of Human Services Child Welfare to make a report. I reviewed the mandatory reporting laws and my obligation to report if a disclosure was received in session. Kelly's mom became tearful, describing her current issue of reporting bruising and marks she has seen when Kelly returned home from parenting time with her father. She had been told by both Child Welfare and the forensic interviewing organization that they did not work with high conflict divorce cases due to the propensity of false allegations and referred her back to Kelly's primary therapist for ongoing care and to review her concerns. I could see the issue this mom was facing and the larger system adding complexity and stress onto Kelly. I told her that I continuously assess for issues related to abuse and trauma and that we would work together if this arose during Kelly's treatment. This is a precarious balance for many clinicians, treating children, who suspect there could be complex dynamics at home.

Assessment

Kelly's mother began bringing her routinely to session. I saw and heard very little from Kelly's father. Finally, Kelly's father sent a message declining to participate altogether as he was busy and referred my contact or questions to Kelly's mother. Kelly's extended assessment drove her treatment planning. Drawing upon the quadripartite trauma assessment, she had individual factors impacting aspects of her development and cognitive state. Kelly presented much younger emotionally and physically than her actual age. She had coping adaptations to perceived adversity which were less than advantageous, but I understood how and why she arrived at her attempts to regulate. Kelly also had various housing changes over the first five years of her life and a complicated medical history. Her medical history included various doctors and specialists all working to solve her gastrointestinal distress, enuresis and encopresis issues. She struggled with peer relationships for several reasons. She needed an intense level of control which stemmed from attachment disruption, temperament and trauma symptoms that she had developed to mitigate hypervigilance. This intensity alienated peers, resulting in arguments and conflict. As peers escalated in conflict so would Kelly; however, her response to a hypervigilant state of distress moved towards aggression and violence until she would literally collapse, often crawling into a ball and crying. Peer relationships were complicated due to attachment behaviors indicating ambivalence and insecurity. Kelly would draw people in and appear to quickly push them away with strong words and impulsive actions. Her medical concerns, with the inability to control elimination, created complications as teachers, school peers or neighborhood children worked to cope with unpleasant smells or accidents during the day. During times of heightened anxiety, both at school and at home, Kelly would smear feces, intensifying the reactions from others.

Kelly was integrated into occupational therapy, pediatric medical care, speech language therapy and now play therapy to support multiple diagnoses, which ranged from elimination and gastrointestinal complications to sensory processing disorder and trauma. She had multiple factors of developmental trauma, high parental ACE measures and symptomatology consistent with transitions of a hyper and hypoaroused state. Her social determinants of health held themes of school and education systems struggling to support her. She had peer group and social skill deficits, low socioeconomic status, insecurity with safety and involvement with various levels of Child Welfare and the legal system. Her family factors indicated a complex structure of high conflict relationship, domestic violence, being isolated as an only child, with parenting practices requiring her to navigate between two very different homes. She was being asked to transition between very different structures, expectations, discipline practices, affect regulation styles, diet, medical support and control. Epigenetic factors included intergenerational trauma effects, setting the stage for instability.

Treatment planning

Individual treatment for Kelly was structured to include directive and non-directive play therapy practices with constructs taken from a neurosequential model utilizing yoga, music with steady rhythm, AATs and play therapy, all entwined or integrated to meet her needs on any given day. Her treatment dovetailed narrative and cognitive constructs with interpersonal neurobiology to form a balanced support enhancing regulation, problem solving and social communication. We planned family sessions to integrate into the individual work utilizing attachment-based theories and filial family therapy with interventions promoting repair to a ruptured attachment relationship. Parent consultations continued to be offered to Kelly's father, with no response; however, her mother routinely attended for psychoeducation, skill building and preparation for family sessions. These family sessions included her incorporating aspects of circle of security and filial work. Kelly connected to play therapy and found both safety and a therapeutic alliance.

The relationship Kelly developed with Apollo was engaging; it included playful exchanges and held opportunities for mastery. Over the next several sessions their relationship solidified, each of them finding attunement within their interactions. As Kelly escalated, so would Apollo, and co-regulation would occur, with my facilitation, to support the process utilizing AANPT. There were several sessions of the "bear in the woods" in which Kelly processed the traumatic death of her grandfather. One session several weeks later, she announced upon entering the playroom:

Kelly: Apollo, we don't need you to guard for the bear! Today we have other things to play.

Apollo: (tilting his head to the side with his tongue hanging out looked at Kelly)

Michelle: Apollo looks interested in what we're going to do today.

Kelly: There is a princess, a castle guard dog and a king and queen.

Michelle: We're ready to hear our parts and play.

Kelly proceeded to find the dress-up clothes needed for the fantasy play. She narrated the script with prompts for what "my lines" were to be. If ever I was unsure of what to say next, I utilized the classic intervention from Gary Landreth of a "stage whisper," with my hand cupped on the side of my mouth in an exaggerated manner. I asked things like, "What should the queen say next?" This session was the start of a new play theme for Kelly; the theme included uncertainty and the idea that people are not always what they seem, you don't know who to trust and you could be hurt at any moment.

There is a dance that occurs in therapy. When a child takes two steps closer towards difficult content, they inherently will take two steps back as a means of remaining balanced within their window of tolerance. Through the fantasy play, ribbons of the child's life weave together, form and take shape, creating a more complete tapestry of their life. Kelly utilized play consistently for several sessions, incorporating a large dragon puppet into the work, which would suddenly leap out and bite me or Apollo. She would narrate harsh words like, "You are a stupid girl! Get into your room God dammit!" and attempt to drag me by the hair to the corner of the playroom. This play required limit-setting self-regulation for me as the co-regulating therapist to avoid us both flooding. I needed to create a continuous holding space for accepting her narrative while maintaining both our physical and emotional safety.

Finally, one afternoon I received a call from her mother. She conveyed through tears and distress that she had picked Kelly up from parenting time. Kelly became clearly distressed upon becoming seat belted in the car and as they drove away began to violently thrash within her seat, removing her seat belt, throwing any objects she could find and attempted to open the car door to get out while the car was still moving. Her mother pulled over the car and began the process she had learned of self-regulation (put your own oxygen mask on first), to co-regulate Kelly. She named the somatic sensation and used describing words for emotions and soothed Kelly through movement and rhythmic song.

Disclosure

Kelly disclosed to her mother in the car her experience with physical and sexual abuse occurring regularly at her father's home. She was able to articulate fear of "dragon breath" and, when asked if she could show her mother what dragon breath looked like, Kelly proceeded to grab her mother's arm and twist violently, hissing words of anger and using adult language and words of shame. She cried, voicing her fear of dragon breath and of being trapped. She had redness on her neck from being choked and she further disclosed her father pressing his fingers inside of her privates or digital penetration of her vagina "when she was bad." This call Kelly's mother made to me resulted in my giving a strong recommendation to the local child welfare office and forensic interviewing team for Kelly to complete forensic interviewing, regardless of the high conflict divorce case. She was seen by the forensic interview team in which her narrative was consistent. Child Welfare services became involved and more medical examinations were arranged to support Kelly in providing testimony for crimes associated with physical and sexual abuse of a child.

Integration

Kelly was a child who utilized movement and storytelling, selecting props when needed to tell her story. She consistently integrated the therapy animal, Apollo, into the process, whether as a source for grounding or to achieve mastery within a given task. Her therapy included themes of low self-worth, grief, losses, guilt and shame associated with the separation from her father, which occurred following her disclosure and subsequent Child Welfare involvement. Although her perception of her father was one in which she felt great pain and sorrow, she continued to love him and blame herself for what happened. Her play included behaviors of repetitious play of abuse and trauma, following the research associated with post-traumatic play.

This play interconnected with behaviors of good people versus bad people, police, court and being jailed. Every week she worked diligently to make sense of her own story and skirted the edges of her window of tolerance towards meaning-making of roles, including who had responsibility to keep kids safe. She grappled with ideas around punishment for those who harm others. Storytelling through role play and dress-up included judges, "bad men" and puppies or babies who became hurt. Puppies or babies in the narrative would receive "dragon breath," be choked or sexually molested and become hurt and confused. Following this re-enactment sequence, Kelly would begin a role play of a criminal trial. Often Apollo was the judge (complete with holding a plastic gavel in his mouth) and I would be in the role of the defense attorney. Kelly would present the case to the judge of what happened, acting as a prosecuting attorney. She was clear about the script when allowed to take the lead and narrated everyone's role. My reflections or statements were designed to be a regulating base for Kelly as she processed through the play and/or to "poke holes in her theory" around victim-blaming through cognitive interweaves. Often, I found my therapeutic role to be one of holding all the aspects of this child's world in one place, helping her remember and reproduce what happened to her. I would mirror the process for Kelly so that she could form connections and tie together her emotional and somatic experience of her autobiography in a meaningful way. During these later play sessions, she engaged in her own regulation with very little input from me. Kelly would pause when she needed and move her body. She used her breath or would stop her feet rhythmically as we had done so often together in the past. She began to need me less and less as she made sense of her history and trauma, integrating the emotional content and narrative within the relationship. The process of coping, regulation and cognition took on an autocatalytic form in which regulation became self-sustaining.

Anna

I (Lindsay) met Anna's mother when she attended an intake session seeking services for her just four-year-old daughter, Anna. I had just started my job as a therapist three weeks before meeting this family. Anna's mother engaged in our biopsychosocial assessment process and reported her daughter had recently disclosed inappropriate touching of Anna by her father. Anna's mother reported that she and Anna's father had divorced early on in Anna's life and the divorce process was tumultuous and "ugly," leading to conflict within the relational dynamic between Anna's parents. Anna's mother described the custody agreement and visitation arrangements and I learned Anna was visiting Dad multiple times per month without supervision. Anna's mother reported she had called Child Welfare and an investigation into Anna's disclosure was underway. She stated Anna's presenting symptoms included a sudden increase in body exploration, nightmares, regression in potty training, peer conflict at school, sudden onset of difficulty separating from Mom at school, and questions regarding whether her father would be picking her up at daycare that seemed to come from a place of anxiety, tearfulness and regression in independence and self-regulatory skills. The mother reported visits were paused while Child Welfare completed their investigation. After the intake I called Child Welfare and made a report to ensure the information I received from the mother was the same information Child Welfare had already received.

I want to take a moment and acknowledge the desire I had, after meeting this family, to find out what happened to this child, to figure out the truth. Throughout this case, I needed a constant internal reminder that it is not my job, and it is not our jobs as therapists, to investigate or "figure out" the truth. Our goal in supporting children therapeutically is to do just that: to meet clients where they are and embark on a journey of processing and redirecting development toward a healthy trajectory. Our only goal is to help the child heal in a manner that allows them to function within their daily lives at a developmentally appropriate level. Oftentimes, parents will come in and ask that we "get a disclosure" from their child. This is not our role. There are many child advocacy centers that engage in forensic interviewing for children and this is where a referral should be sent, should a parent's goal for therapy be to gain a disclosure. It is vital to the process to clarify roles early in the therapeutic relationship should a parent's goal be centered around getting a disclosure of abuse or neglect.

I met Anna the following week at her first appointment with me. I introduced myself and let her know I had spent some time talking to her Mom the week prior. She presented as shy and unsure about interacting with me initially and didn't say much. I invited Anna and her mother back to my playroom to help ease the transition and let Anna have a safe base from which to explore this new environment. Anna entered the playroom and her eyes lit up upon seeing a literal room full of toys. She whispered something in her mom's ear, her mom nodded enthusiastically, and Anna left Mom's side to begin exploring the playroom. I followed Anna at a distance so not to invade her space and verbally "introduced" her to the toys she was looking at as she walked along the shelves. Anna stopped at the sandtray and I narrated her actions in the sandtray. She ran her hands through the sand and I let her know that she could put anything on the shelves behind her into the sandtray. She picked a few items out and engaged me in a game of hide and seek with small items in the sandtray. I observed her attempting to cover her smiles and stifle her giggles and excitement throughout my attempts at finding the objects she had hidden. She asked to switch roles, so I could hide objects for her. Shortly after, she called her mother over and suggested we play pretend that it was her birthday, she was a princess, and we must make her multiple birthday cakes and hide her birthday presents while she slept. I did not realize it at the time, but after reflecting upon this case in supervision, I noticed this moment was where her post-traumatic play began.

Over the next few sessions Anna no longer needed her mother in session to help her regulate. She was able to separate from her mother and enter individual sessions enthusiastically, leading the session as if it were second nature. She continued engaging in the play sequence that included her as a princess celebrating her birthday, and I was required to make birthday cakes and hide gifts. Slowly but surely her play began to shift. She began asking me to be the queen while she was the princess, and her play began to include moments where we would be in danger, suddenly, in the middle of her typical play sequence. The reason for the danger was vague initially, and we were never able to get out of danger despite my attempts as "the queen" to ensure safety. We ran around the room in our princess dresses and crowns, hiding from the danger for weeks on end. I continually assessed for shifts in the play sequence, but we seemed stuck. Eventually, I decided to engage in a more robust manner within the play sequence. The next session we carried on with our usual play sequence and when we became stuck and unable to flee from danger I reflected, "I feel so scared, we keep trying to get away, but we just can't! I think we need help!" Anna played along and stated her princess's friends were coming to save us from the "bad guys." She grabbed my Disney princess miniatures off my sandtray shelves and had them punch and kick the "bad guys," which she envisioned in my bop bag. I reacted with shock and awe at the courage and strength of these princesses and reflected as much to Anna. The princesses defeated the "bad guys" and saved the day.

Throughout this process I integrated moments in the sessions where I would name how I felt about the intensity of the play sequence and apply a developmentally appropriate coping skill to model and encourage identification of a feeling and application of a coping skill. One day, Anna came in and reported she was not interested in her princess play and wanted to do something different. I let her know it was her choice as she walked slowly through the room looking at the various items around my room. She paused at a poster depicting a child doing a variety of yoga poses and asked, "Do you know yoga?" We had a conversation and I reminded her of my certification as a children's yoga instructor and she responded with excitement and enthusiasm and told me that she does yoga at her school. She then asked to do some yoga, so I sat with her and asked her to choose a narrative from the one of our yoga curriculums. She chose a narrative that takes place in a castle with kings, queens, knights and horses and donned her usual pink princess dress. I began leading her through the narrative, modeling poses as we went. Shortly after starting, Anna suggested I read the story to her while she chose the poses we would do. I agreed, and she took charge of the rest of the session. After this session, Anna would randomly switch between engaging in her post-traumatic play sequence and requesting a session in which we did yoga. After looking over Anna's notes, I became aware that it seemed as though she would spend five or six sessions in her post-traumatic play sequence and abruptly shift to yoga in an attempt to disconnect from her trauma processing and regulate. After regulating, she would be able to re-engage in her post-traumatic play sequence, often with significant shifts in play occurring immediately after a session of yoga. It is important to point out that Anna's father had not reached out to Anna's mother regarding visits after the Child Welfare investigation concluded. We continued to engage in therapeutic sessions to process her trauma, as well as the grief, loss and confusion Anna struggled with regarding the lack of contact from her father.

Our play patterns continued this way for a few months until one day when Anna came in and began her usual post-traumatic play sequence. She was dressed as a princess and was walking to retrieve the sandtray princesses once again. She stopped in her tracks after getting the princesses and ran over to my dramatic play materials. She grabbed a Halloween costume that had a Superman symbol on the chest and a red skirt attached to it and brought it to me. She requested I put it on her. "OK," I said, "but you might need to get out of the princess dress, so it will fit." Anna adamantly refused and requested that I figure out a way to put the Superman costume on over her dress because she needed both. I somehow managed to get it on her over the large pink tulle gown. "I'm a princess that is also a superhero, but that part's secret," she said. She was, indeed, a tiny, lumpy version of a superhero. "You are a princess and a superhero," I said. "What do we do now?" Anna re-entered the play sequence with no other shifts to her play this session. As time went on, wearing the superhero costume over the princess dress became part of her post-traumatic play. After a few weeks and another yoga session, she reported the sandtray princesses were now her "sidekicks" and, though she was a superhero princess, they were there to help save her because she could not quite do it completely on her own.

I have a little co-therapist, a French bulldog named Olive. I integrated her into the work using animal assisted play therapy sessions with a neurobiologically informed model after I received post-graduate training in animal assisted human health and Olive received extensive training and vetting as a therapy dog. Anna met Olive about five months after her intake session. Anna integrated Olive into her post-traumatic play sequence seamlessly. "We need a trap," she said. She created a trap out of two stacked hula hoops and a long Play-Doh "snake" on the art table and requested that Olive be placed inside the trap. "Pretend that Olive is my dog and the bad guy stole her and wants to hurt her." Olive, always up for playtime, jumped right onto the table and into the pretend trap. Anna then shifted her play again and, for the first time, decided to take on the bad guys herself, with the help of her "sidekicks" – about 30 sandtray miniatures including the princesses, feelings characters from *Inside Out*, ponies, superheroes, fairies, unicorns and other fantastic, friendly-appearing characters. As you can imagine, this setup took a significant amount of time of our session just to prepare. We often had to end sessions before we were able to move past the initial setup.

Anna disconnected from her setup process to engage in a few sessions of yoga. Initially, it appeared she had regressed as she began struggling to separate from her mother at the beginning of sessions and would request her mother engage in yoga with us as well. Anna always requested the yoga narrative be filled with princesses, queens, kings, castles and dragons and, as her post-traumatic play sequence shifted, so did her yoga process. She began by getting dressed in her princess dress, taking off her shoes and setting up the child-sized yoga mats. Anna directed me and her mother to engage in yoga while she led us through the narrative. She assigned us roles, with Mom as queen, Anna as princess, and I was the princess's sister. Anna led us through her memory of the yoga narrative, shifting the intensity and details to fit what felt right to her. Anna utilized yoga and created her own yoga "poses" during the sessions she led, and after a few weeks of yoga, Anna was ready to re-engage in play.

Anna returned to session with a motivation I had not seen before. She sped into my office declaring we had a lot of work to do. Anna kicked off her shoes, got into the usual princess dress and the superhero outfit, grabbed the "traps" and began setting up her side-kicks around the trap. She coaxed Olive into the trap, handed me a small container of bug miniatures and told me I was the "bad guy" and directed me to throw the bugs toward Olive. Anna ran to the other side of my room, jumped on my couch and pretended to be asleep. "Pretend I'm asleep and you're the bad guy and I wake up because my dog is missing," she said, "but I don't wake up until you throw the bugs at Olive." "Alright," I said, unsure of how I felt about throwing tiny plastic bugs at my dog. I gently tossed single bugs at Olive who looked at me, confused, while she stood in the trap. I threw in a wicked laugh and commented that I was going to "get" the dog. Anna jumped up off the couch immediately and ran at me full force. She screamed at the top of her lungs and pushed me with all her might. "YOU CAN'T HURT MY PUPPY!" she said. She then began punching and kicking me as hard as her little body would let her while continuing to yell. It is important to note, Anna was, and I'm sure still is, a kind, thoughtful, intelligent child who often struggled to stand up for herself amongst her peers. Anna would come to session regularly with reports of peers bullying her and struggled consistently to ask teachers for help or stand up for herself. The aggression Anna demonstrated this session was definitely not a typical behavior or mindspace for Anna. "Woah!" I said. "You are so angry!" Anna snapped out of her aggression instantly, looked up at me, seemingly shocked at the interaction, and apologized. I reassured her it was OK and validated the big feelings she was experiencing. The very next session Anna disclosed her sexual abuse experience to me.

After her disclosure, Anna would vacillate between engaging in her post-traumatic play sequence, yoga and engaging in expressive therapies to process her experience as well as the grief and loss that came with trying to make sense of her relationship with her dad. I could tell when Anna became dysregulated during her sessions, because she would often resort to targeted physical aggression toward me while processing. Anna would grab a shark miniature off the shelves and bring it close to my face and have it "bite" my cheek by pinching its mouth closed on my cheek as hard as she could. Her post-traumatic play sequence shifted, and she started sessions by skipping trap setup altogether and instead saving Olive and vanquishing the "bad guy" with swords, fists and feet. It is important to point out that

I struggled in this moment to make a clinical decision regarding both my safety and Anna's therapeutic process. I was a brand new therapist and, though I was able to see the therapeutic benefit of being a literal punching bag for Anna once a week, I also didn't particularly enjoy it and was concerned about reinforcing the idea that aggression toward others was socially acceptable. Thankfully, after lots of thinking and a few supervision sessions, I was able to shift the bad guy to a more appropriate item, my bop bag. Anna took to my introduction of the bop bag as the bad guy for aggression instantly. I remained in the role of the bad guy up until the point of aggression, and Anna would run to the bop bag and strike it repeatedly, while screaming "You can't hurt her! It's not OK!" Occasionally Anna would be so intensely involved in her post-traumatic play she would forget to utilize the bop bag and require some redirection. However, Anna was a fast learner and was able to make the shift without any detriment or significant change to her therapeutic process. As a new therapist, this experience helped me learn that it is possible to set limits while honoring and meeting your client where they are in their therapeutic process. I am forever grateful for this lesson, as it has helped me scaffold treatment for many clients I have had the pleasure of working with after meeting Anna.

Throughout my nearly two years with Anna I incorporated multiple expressive therapies such as therapeutic art, narrative therapy, music therapy, movement, yoga and play therapy to ensure she was processing through multiple mediums. Anna hit some significant barriers to continued processing, usually due to typical developmental hindrances in her ability to conceptualize abstract thought, but she was always able to push through. A year and a half after I started seeing Anna, her father re-entered the picture and requested visits once again. Anna's mother refused visits and filed an emergency custody change with the court. I was subpoenaed to testify in the family court proceeding and the result of the hearing was the addition of significant limitations on the father's unsupervised visitations with Anna. During the hearing the father refused to see Anna altogether due to these limitations. I continued seeing Anna to help her process the continued disconnection from her father and paternal family, in addition to her trauma. Over time, she began presenting more and more like a typical five-year-old child. She began maintaining well in her educational environment and reported she had been dreaming solely about "rainbows and unicorns flying through the sky" when I asked her ongoing assessment questions around nightmares and sleep issues. Her post-traumatic play dwindled away and soon her play lacked intensity. Eventually, when Anna came into session it felt as though we were "just playing," rather than engaging in play with a purpose other than having fun. Anna and I terminated our therapeutic relationship. I recently received a card from her family and it appears she is doing well. It is my most sincere hope that she is able to safely re-engage with her father one day, as healthy parent–child relationships are vital to the social–emotional development of children.

Anna taught me a lot, as one of my first sexual abuse cases. She taught me about the resilience of children and families, neuroplasticity, micro fashion, the power of movement, play and humor, diversity in expression of emotions and the importance of meeting children where they are and trusting in their process. Her family taught me about the importance of holding space for each family member involved in a childhood trauma case and taking their culture, needs and life experiences into consideration when treating their smallest members. I am humbled and honored to have worked with Anna and her family.

Incorporating sandtray into yoga and play therapy practices

Dr. Margaret Lowenfeld was the first psychotherapist to use sand as a tool for treatment with children. During the late 1920s she turned from physical medicine towards psychotherapeutic care, finding new tools to help access the child's subconscious and inner world. She titled the sandplay after H.G. Wells's book *Floor Games* and introduced small toys which children could use to create stories, with scenes that were realistic or fantastical. During the mid-twentieth century, Dora Kalff viewed the world of floorgames technique through a Jungian psychotherapeutic lens and developed sandplay. Sandplay differs in form, function and facilitation from sandtray therapies, although even today the two types of sand work can become confused by practitioners (Klaff 1988). Sandtray is a specialized process within play therapy or therapeutic arts which introduces the tactile process of sand in conjunction with a selection of miniatures to symbolically represent the client's thought process or experience. Homeyer and Sweeney (2011, p.4) define sandtray *therapy* as:

> an expressive and projective mode of psychotherapy involving the unfolding and processing of intra and interpersonal issues through the use of specific sandtray materials as a nonverbal medium of communication, led by the client(s) and facilitated by a trained therapist.

We often describe to artistically anxious clients that sandtray is a way to create art without having to worry about whether you're a "good artist." This often puts clients at ease and opens the door of possibility for utilizing art as a way of self-expression. Gisela Schubach De Domenico once discussed a child participant of sandtray in her work, describing the type of therapy as helping a thinking process unfold. The picture in the sand becomes thought that you can see more clearly (Schubach De Domenico 1988). The Jungian approach relies on the unconscious communication with the psyche using symbol as the language of archetypes. Thus, the representation created in the sand is translated into the archetypal human language; usually a therapist is not teaching the client this language but holding their translations silently.

Sandtray has value in a variety of ways. It provides expression to non-verbalized thought or emotional processes, has a unique kinesthetic quality, serves to create a necessary therapeutic distance for children, provides a safe holding environment for trauma processing, is effective for clients experiencing adversity, is inclusive experientially and provides boundaries and limits promoting relational safety (Homeyer and Sweeney 2011). Sandtray experiences typically include offering a wet and dry sand option; however, some children with sensory processing issues or who have sensitivities may have strong opinions regarding one sand type or another. Variety and options are what is important for a play therapy setting. Sandtray requires a wide range of miniatures for selection to allow children options for representing experience. The selection of materials is captured in the work of Gisela Schubach De Domenico (1988) in which she states miniatures need to have imagery that comes to life, including the earth, minerals, plants, animal and human kingdoms. We are not collecting at random, but selecting miniatures that represent all aspects of humanity and experience. Therefore it is important to select figures that repel you in addition to those that draw you in, select miniatures that bore you, some that appear tasteless, horrifying, evil, good, magical, harmonious and some that strike you as downright absurd (Schubach De Domenico 1988).

Categories of miniatures with a few examples therapists often find useful to include are:

Family groups: spanning cultures, socioeconomic status, lifespan, emotions, etc.

Animals: wild animals, domestic animals, prehistoric, rural life (farm), aquatic

"Creepy crawlies": insects, snakes, bugs, arachnids

People: spanning occupations, sexuality, gender, athletics, historical figures and religious figures

Buildings and structures: a wide range of houses, buildings, bridges, caves, cages, civil structures, religious structures, historical structures and mystical structures

Movement: transportation items, helicopters, airplanes, trains, cars, trucks, buses, boats, rocket ships

Natural: rocks, moss, plants, trees, sea shells (we have luck finding miniatures not only in our natural world but from aquatic stores selling fish tank art and supplies)

Fences/gates/doors: barriers and fences of a variety of types, doors (dollhouse supply stores can be helpful here), arches, gates, enclosures

Magical and mystical: wizards, fairies, demons, cauldrons, wishing wells, dragons, unicorns, Pegasus, gargoyles, Cerberus (and other folklore from Greek and Roman mythology), movie characters

Scary: monsters, ghosts, skeletons, beasts, etc.

Illness: syringe props, medicine bottles, empty plastic pill cases, medical toys

Furniture/household: dollhouse furniture, tools, food, electronic devices

Alcohol/substances: miniature wine bottles, small alcohol bottles (syringe prop, medicine bottles often used)

Death and dying: gravestones, coffins, religious figures, doctors, nurses

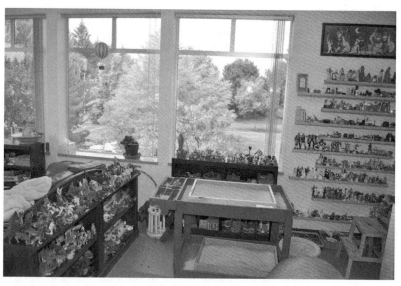

*Figure 3.4 Example of a sandtray with miniatures
for creative expression in play therapy*

Sandtray can utilize directive and non-directive approaches, can incorporate a variety of theoretical frameworks or can integrate several theories, allowing the client the ability to create a symbolic representation of their experience. The therapist generally reflects the shared experience of the sandtray in relationship with the client (Kestly 2015). This can include verbal or non-verbal cues. For example, if the client has chosen, let's say a dragon and a puppy, and the feelings in the room have become very intense and need regulating, the therapist may say something like, "the dragon is so big and the puppy is so small, but I see helpers in front of him and he is inside this house"; or the therapist may simply use their body, breath and nonverbal cues to visibly regulate the emotion. The physical movement drawing upon yoga philosophy of deep, audible breaths, stretch and/or slight swaying or rocking indicates there has been intensity and the therapist is regulating, which in turn will co-regulate the child.

Emily

Six-year-old Emily was in treatment due to child sexual abuse. Emily was referred to treatment by the forensic interview team. She had symptoms including sudden crying, voicing feelings of guilt, shame and self-blame, sleep disturbances including nightmares and fear of the dark, school difficulties (fidgety, up and down in her seat, needing to use the bathroom frequently, poor concentration), withdrawal from friends, lack of appetite, anxiety and fear of separation from her mother. Emily entered into treatment and was drawn to sandtray and utilized it throughout her process. She naturally included movement throughout her experience to titrate emotions. This was further developed through yoga narratives later in treatment. Emily never spoke directly of her abuse experience; however, she created her trauma narrative through symbolic play. She inherently knew, within her own wisdom, that movement was needed to shift from a state of dysregulation back to a regulated state. The window of tolerance is a theory to represent boundaries which hold the various intensities of emotional arousal of an individual. Movement beyond these boundaries disrupts thinking and behavior; however, regulated states, which remain within the boundaries, allow for thinking and connection of ideas to occur (Siegel 2012). This theory base was visible within Emily's sessions. Many children who have been abused have already moved through a process of intense forensic interviewing, and Emily happened to have been in this position. It wasn't important therapeutically for her to verbally specify the who, what, when, where, why of the abuse. This wasn't necessary for her therapy, nor was it my role. Instead, our treatment goals included integration of the experiences to find meaning, to build mastery to result in empowerment. Symbolic play and movement provide the ability for a whole-body approach to treatment. Words alone cannot necessarily process and integrate a trauma experience for a child; however, expressive arts provide opportunity for the mind and body to connect the emotional and sensory knowledge of the experience.

Emily was also a child who needed time to build rapport within the playroom. She spent three sessions utilizing free play, exploring the room and deciding if I (Michelle) was safe. As mentioned above, children who come to me following the disclosure of abuse may have already been through a series of forensic interviews, as well as having had involvement with various authorities such as local police and the Department of Human Services (DHS). It is not uncommon for parents to "prep" their children for therapy by saying I'm a "feelings doctor" or that they are going to a special place to be able to talk about what happened. We might be able to imagine what it would be like to be six years old and told by someone you love and care about that you're going to see a new person in a new strange place who has toys and supposedly "doctors the feelings up." This experience is one in which a child understands that they are expected to talk about the most frightening, scary, intimate, confusing experience of their life. Understandably, Emily entered the playroom during those first three sessions cautiously. I explained that I understood why her mom brought her to see me and that this was a room where she got to choose…everything. She could say whatever she needed to say, do whatever she needed to do, and I was there to listen. I told Emily I might have questions, but she could choose whether or not to answer them and if she answered them, she could choose to do so through words or by showing me. I explained that is what all of the toys were for (hands sweeping across the room); here you get to show me and can use as few or as many toys as you like if you don't want to tell me with words. The choices are always yours and this is a place you can't get in trouble no matter what happens.

Emily proceeded during those first three sessions to thoroughly test that introduction. During her first session she proceeded to make the biggest mess of all messes, checking in throughout to see my reaction. "I can't get in trouble, I can make a mess." I reflected back that if she needed a mess, then we needed to make a mess. Emily smiled and said, "Alright, let's clean this up." We laughed, and she talked about her pets at home while she cleaned and arranged toys. Emily used her next session, for lack of better words, to test strong or offensive language. She specifically used sexual language in addition to announcing "all the bad words she knew." All the while, Emily looked at my face to see what reaction would be there. I reacted authentically: "Wow! That is a strong word" and "We get to say it in here if we need to." It was important that she didn't get a false reaction. The language was strong, we could use it and not get in trouble; however, to react stoically would have been incongruent with the situation. The third session she began to scan the room and ask questions about "other kids." "Do other kids use these nerf guns?" "Do the other kids that come here play with these toys?" I responded by normalizing the situation. "Kids come to see me for all sorts of reasons, often when something has happened, and they need a space to think and play with someone who can listen." She nodded solemnly and proceeded to organize the dollhouse. I reflected how sometimes organizing things helped me think and calm down my worries. She simply glanced up at me and worked in silence.

The fourth session, Emily selected what I attributed during the remainder of her treatment as being a perpetrator symbol. Paris Goodyear-Brown (2010, p.14) describes perpetrator symbols as "any miniature, puppet, art creation or other toy that the child may choose to represent the person or people who hurt him." Emily selected a large black dragon during this session:

Emily: This is bad and needs to be locked away.

Michelle: (responding with a big audible breath) His mouth is open, I can't tell if he is growling, smiling or trying to say something, but this is bad.

Emily: He's smiling because he knows he is going to do bad things and make you feel yucky.

Michelle: I just felt my stomach…it feels like there is a knot tied up.

Emily: Me too. I feel sick (Emily put the dragon in the sand and bent her body over sitting down).

Michelle: Maybe I can stretch this out and breathe a little (I mirrored Emily's movement, but moved into a "cat pose").

Emily: (also moving into a "cat pose" began to make a cat noise) Rrrroooowwww!

Michelle: (made the cat noises back)

Emily: (moved into "hero pose" on her own, a natural position for her and smiled) He needs to go away.

Michelle: He needs to go away, let's find a place for him to go.

Emily: (picking up the dragon) You're bad! RRRROOOOWWWW! (shouting her cat noise in the dragon's face) I'm now going to tie him up.

Michelle: You're going to find something to tie him up with.

Emily: Yup (Emily found a jump rope and proceeded to tie the dragon up). He can't see now which feels super scary. You can only feel what happens to you, but you can't see anything.

This was the first session that Emily began moving into her trauma narrative through symbolic play.

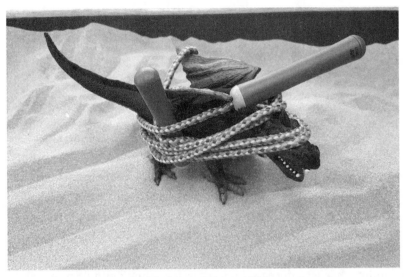

Figure 3.5 Emily's dragon tied up with his eyes covered

Emily: (looked at the dragon intensely) He could still get away.

Michelle: (reflecting the emotion) This still doesn't feel safe.

Emily: (grabbed a wooden cage to contain the dragon) There, he's trapped and now we're going to be OK.

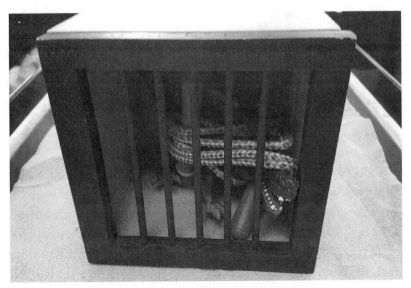

Figure 3.6 Emily's dragon further contained in a cage

Michelle: (reflection back with authenticity) He's tied up and locked in this cage. I didn't realize I was holding my breath.

Emily: Me too!

Michelle: (I take a full yoga breath)

Emily: (takes a full yoga breath)

Emily's trauma narrative continued through use of the sandtray metaphor and symbolic play infused with movement and the inclusion of yoga. She slowly put the pieces together of her sexual abuse history, including being blindfolded for much of her experience. Emily's perpetrator was a grandfather, whom she used to spend time with when her parents were traveling for business. Her grandmother was deceased and therefore she would be alone with her grandfather for days at a time. Family members perpetrating child sexual abuse crimes are not uncommon, with approximately 40 percent of sexual abuse cases being attributed to family members (Gaskill and Perry 2012). Intrafamilial sexual abuse creates further complexity, as children often expect family figures, such as parents, grandparents, uncles or aunts, to be protective or sources of comfort; the abuse yields confusion and disruption to attachment patterns (Gil 2006). Emily had been told a series of lies, including things like grandfathers and granddaughters get to have special playtime and she couldn't tell because if she did he would get sick and maybe die. What became critically important for Emily was the strong support she experienced following disclosure throughout the judicial process. The complexity of emotions experienced by the family system was intense and division within the system occurred as a result. However, her mother and father both believed and supported her. Emily also found herself surrounded by what she later symbolically called her "lady guardians," and represented them with miniatures of warrior princesses, powerful fairies and nurturing figures. These women were the police detectives working her case; the forensic interviewer (also female), her mother, her aunt and myself were represented as powerful allies. Emily consistently chose a large bear, which represented her father, and a small spotted fawn to represent herself. These types of symbols can represent a child's need to see themselves as powerful or vulnerable, and a variety of other dispositions, depending upon the child's history and perception of self. Sometimes transitional objects come from home and children who bring a "special toy," "stuffy" or "lovey" from their home may be bringing a symbolic representation of their attachment figure or secure base (Winnicott 1953). These should never be discounted or set aside or the child discouraged from bringing it back to the playroom. Children bring what is needed from home and therapists can incorporate these objects into the therapeutic process, either through symbolic play or to assist in regulation.

Emily created a sandtray during a session that moved through confusion and a variety of complex emotions, often associated with intrafamilial sexual abuse, and ended with an embodied state of mastery and empowerment. Emily, always remaining in metaphor and symbolic play, told the story of the fawn and the dragon. The lady guardians protected the fawn along with the "big papa bear." No dragon could get to the fawn because Emily stated the baby deer was loved and important.

Emily: Baby deer are not for hurting. You cannot touch the baby deer again!

Michelle: The baby deer is in here (pointing inside the police station) and there are lots of things outside of the entrance.

Emily: The police and the entire army protect this baby deer. She is loved and important.

Michelle: This baby deer knows how important she is and that she is surrounded by the people who believed her and love her.

Emily: The dragon is laying down and cries like a little baby. He knows he is bad.

Michelle: The dragon is laying down and crying. This picture feels both sad and glad, seeing the dragon laying down and crying.

Emily: Yes…the dragon was not always bad. These tigers (pointing at some of the guardians representing family members) are mad and sad and glad.

Michelle: That sounds like it would be confusing to have so many mixed up feelings.

Emily: The dragon has mixed up feelings, the papa bear and baby deer have mixed up feelings too. It is sad and good he is crying. (Emily leaves the sandtray and begins flailing her arms)

Michelle: These mixed up feelings feel really big. My body feels it too (I flail my arms to match and then begin to move them more fluidly into an airplane pose).

Emily: (moves her arms and begins to "fly around the room") RRRROOOOWWWW! (shouts her cat noise from a previous session)

Michelle: RRRROOOOWWWW! (matching the intensity and shifting into slower purring noise)

Emily: (begins to cry and sits down on the floor)

Michelle: I'm here with you (sits down nearby).

Emily: (gets up and moves back to the sandtray; she moves the deer outside of the police station, grabs a guardian miniature to join the deer and they both march next to the dragon; the deer remains between two guardians facing the dragon) I loved you and you were bad to me! My heart feels broken and I'm mad at you! (naturally moves into a new posture, which is also known through yoga physical poses as a star pose)

Michelle: I think the dragon can hear her (mirrors star pose). She is using a strong and powerful voice.

Emily: (moves back to a standing position and looks at the dragon) I think you know you were wrong now. We are going to be OK without you.

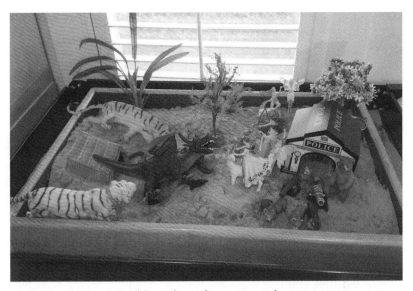

Figure 3.7 Emily's sandtray of protection and empowerment

Emily's play shifted at that point, moving forward toward themes of empowerment with a physical nature of an integrated and regulated state. She used movement and breath along with a narrative storytelling to describe girls who were strong, smart and surrounded by friends and people who loved them.

CHAPTER 4

Yoga and Play Can Happen in Every Setting

GROUP AND FAMILY SYSTEMS

Family play and yoga therapy

Sometimes our professional worlds appear split. Therapists can feel like they are either in one branch of work or another. The world of social work often sees this divide, meaning you are either considered to be a micro or a macro social work practitioner. The professional world of therapy can experience a division such as either practicing with children individually or from a family therapy perspective. I often wonder why we can't do it all whenever possible? Stepping outside of the direct clinical or micro setting into macro level policy issues provides opportunities for us to become advocates for what brings the children we work with into our offices, thus working toward larger system or political change to create lasting impacts on future generations of children. Stepping outside of the individual therapy experiences and into the family context allows a systems perspective to unfold. Therefore we create change in the system which the child is embedded within. The authors believe that, whenever possible, treatment planning needs to include all aspects of the child's world with intervention for every system possible, creating change which is autocatalytic or self-sustaining.

The field of family therapy is rooted within the social work movement. General systems theory closely considers the interactions and relationships among all parts of the family system. Family therapy is viewed through this lens: the family being an independent system comprised of multiple subsystems in which the whole of the family is greater than the sum of its parts (individual members) (Patterson *et al.* 2009). Systems theory emphasizes relationships, interactional patterns, influences, power and roles among members of the system (McGoldrick 1999). This perspective includes the context of larger systems (political, community, government programs, etc.) which all impact the family and individual members. The concept of homeostasis permeates this model, meaning a family will seek equilibrium during times of rupture, fluctuation or change. The equilibrium of a family system may be perceived by an outsider as being unbalanced, chaotic or unhealthy; however, for that family, it is a balanced state. All the individual parts of the system work to maintain the state of equilibrium. It is not uncommon to see one family member improve in functioning, health, introspective awareness or gain insight, thus changing behavior, and a different family member "fall apart" or assume behaviors which place the family back in their original state of equilibrium. The practice we have discussed considers offering wrap-around support whenever possible to all members of the family. This can be in the form of a sibling or multiple siblings gaining access to care, adult individual counseling and/or couple support when needed, to ensure we are reaching the entire system while facilitating the change process.

Family play and yoga therapy will most often include structured play therapy in which the therapist takes an active role to determine the session content and course of therapy that given day. Non-directive play therapy sessions can occur within a family context; however, this can create opportunity for chaos to unfold as you increase the number of family members. We will more often see non-directive play sessions with parent–child dyads as a means for the therapist to assess and participate when needed within a parent–child play interaction theory including attachment or filial-based models.

The concept of integrating touch and movement into family therapy is not new. Virginia Satir, in her experiential approach to therapy, encouraged touch between parents and their children and used playful activities including role play or family sculpts (Axline 1969; Duhl, Kantor and Duhl 1973). This includes family members showing physical and symbolic relationships. The emotional system, often implicit within family communication, was a goal of Satir's, with the intention of every family member finding ownership in "the problem" that has brought the child to therapy. This helps open a window of possibility towards change within the larger system, not scapegoating a child into taking full responsibility for dysfunction. Touch and movement within the context of family therapy was again brought to our awareness through attachment-based interventions such as Theraplay® (Booth and Jernberg 2009; Munns 2011) in which the therapist actively works with the family through use of therapeutic touch and relational interactions, mirroring that of early mother/baby experiences to repair attachment relationships.

Integrating movement in the form of yoga builds not only upon the philosophical underpinnings of yoga but entwines family therapy and systems concepts. We can incorporate yoga movement into building genograms with children. Yoga and forms of movement have been incorporated into our family therapy sessions. All members of the family can be present for a session when completing a play genogram through introduction of yoga. Pictures of yoga poses which provide clear direction and demonstrate poses are helpful to family members, especially for those for whom yoga is a novel concept. We also open the possibility for any posture, pose or body structure in these interventions, as we don't want creativity or symbolism to be limited to yoga poses or the cards provided. This is like the process of a family play genogram miniature selection, in which we may have family members choose from miniatures or any object within the entire play therapy room. This is expanded again by offering clay or other media for creating a representation if what is needed cannot be found.

Drawing upon knowledge and work of family sculptures you can use yoga poses as a means of communicating roles, relationship or connections among subgroups within the system. These movements can also indicate patterns or highlight how the family maintains equilibrium. Utilizing partner poses can aid in this and tell a family's story or move towards repair within an attachment relationship. Yoga poses can become integrated in creating family constellations, drawing upon family systems theory to better understand present or past experiences, adversity and how a family may be coping or adjusting to transition and/or trauma such as grief work, divorce within the system or alcoholism and parental mental health illness. Creating a family narrative includes bringing the yoga to life, adding narratives and creative storytelling to the process. Creative storytelling, utilizing yoga and play, offers this intervention as a means for every member of the family to participate in the therapy process including the youngest and oldest. The methodology works well with highly intellectualized family members as we are creating opportunity for "heady" family members to leave a highly analytical zone and move into their body through somatosensory experience, allowing emotion to take form and shape within the process. This storytelling can follow the guidelines and practice principles outlined through the family puppet interview described below.

Family yoga interview

How can we act out a narrative using our body to tell a story? This concept builds upon the work seen within family therapy and through the intervention utilizing puppets and narrative storytelling termed the *family puppet interview*. Integrating yoga, drawing from the eight limbs of practice, can offer opportunity for both regulation and creativity of body movement through dramatization of the narrative. The clinician can gather associations to the material presented by "interviewing" the yoga poses (Irwin and Malloy 1975), thus staying within the metaphor. We ask families to utilize the yoga postures or, if one is not available, to utilize creativity by finding a new character which represents their narrative (we saw Kelly do this on her own by changing one posture into the name of another to include a penguin and a dragon in her story).

Gil (2015) describes asking families to create a story with a beginning, middle and an end. The story is to be of their own creation and not a replication of a favorite fairy tale, television show or movie. The family can choose the number of yoga poses needed and then act out the narrative using movement and narration of their character(s). We ask the family to stay in character and narrate the story from that character's perspective, rather than narrating from a "classic narrator" perspective. For example, instead of narrating "the cat arches her back because she is frightened by all this noise," the family member would act out the sequence "aaahh, I'm frightened by all this noise and need to arch my back to show all of you that I feel scared."

Not only are these stories often insightful, but the process of creating the story provides valuable data to the therapist on how the family functions, which roles predominate in the family, personality types and problem solving techniques during mild stress or pressure. We ask the family to spend a little time going through yoga cards and/or thinking of what they would like to be within the story. They may need some "warm up time" to get into poses and movements and also may ask for assistance in gaining the "correct posture." Our response is often, "Your posture will be what feels most comfortable in your body or is needed for your story; we don't need to worry in here about all our movements being correct." This may need to be reiterated to some parents who struggle to move out of a "teaching" role with their child and to accept the child's movements or posture being correct...even when it is not a perfect plank pose and lands somewhere between plank and downward dog.

These activities can be disarming for families and result in un-expected outcomes. I (Michelle) remember after one session in particular with two highly intellectual and skeptical parents (one held a medical degree and the other a doctorate of philosophy in engineering), both parents turned toward one another and the mother stated: "I had no idea that this is what would come from 'make up a story with a beginning, middle and an end'..." They both laughed, and the father said, "Well, I can see why you have the degree in this. We clearly have some work to do and are ready to get started. What comes next."

Finding creative methods of incorporating the right hemisphere of the brain through music, movement, dance, drama, art and play is what we consider the key for helping families facing adverse life experiences and trauma. The expressive arts methods allow for full integration, creating cohesive narratives and understanding with meaning-making, allowing families to find new opportunities for change.

Group work: using yoga, AANPT and play therapy with groups of children

Group play integrated into yoga offers an opportunity to neuro-sequentially move through difficult content in the context of a community relationship. Group play interventions are dynamic and help support fundamental social skills, life skills and the ability to be seen and accepted by peers. The group process provides a "like-me" phenomenon, creating opportunity for children to not feel alone in their cancer diagnosis, paternal or maternal alcoholism, divorce, grief or abuse. Drawing upon the knowledge outlined in Chapter 1, we can see the power of play as a therapeutic agent of change in group work. Research regarding group therapy has consistently demonstrated the effectiveness of child and adolescent group work (Abramowitz 1976; Beeferman and Orvaschel 1994; Sweeney, Baggerly and Ray 2014).

Group work is dynamic and does require training to facilitate and navigate ethical components associated with group processes, and to understand engaging in clinical practice with multi-cultural competency. If facilitating a group in which you are incorporating play and yoga practices, it is important to ensure your informed consent reflects risks associated with confidentiality during a shared process and risks associated with movement and emotional discomfort that may be associated with processing difficult content areas. Below we have outlined the rationale and first two weeks of curriculum for a children's divorce group incorporating yoga and play. The principles used to create the narrative we describe have been applied to other presenting issues, but therapists can utilize this concept and create their own unique or original curricula building upon this work.

Group work for children experiencing divorce using yoga and play therapy

Adverse childhood experiences span many and various aspects of early trauma or attachment disruptions. Divorce is one adverse experience that can be incorporated into a group setting. Yoga is an innovative practice to decrease symptomatology associated with a dysregulated nervous system. Yoga treats somatic issues such as stress, anxiety or hyperarousal (Galantino, Galhavy and Quinn 2008). Dovetailing yoga with play therapy within a group process forms the foundation for connection and safety, thus increasing regulation and creating the ability for cognitive restructuring of adverse events such as divorce. If we look back to Chapter 2, Kelly's family had been court-ordered to attend a divorce group that included psychoeducation as the primary factor. This isn't uncommon, as many judges now require divorcing or legally separating parents with children under the age of seventeen to attend parent education programs with the intended aim of reducing child distress and improving adjustment (Galovan and Schramm 2017). The current model for providing children with support during divorce or parental separation lies squarely in psychoeducation as the platform, administered classroom style, with brief time for questions and group discussion. The yoga and play framework combines movement and expressive arts and is constructed with the understanding of attachment theory, primarily how divorce negatively impacts the attachment relationship (Fraley and Heffernan 2012). Parenting styles are considered, along with current neuroscience and trauma theory, including the neurosequential model of therapeutics (Perry 2006). This application uses child yoga and play therapy, adding a concrete element of understanding to include practice experience for robust outcomes which align with learning and developmental theories (Carey *et al.* 2015). To ask a child to process what may be a traumatic experience associated with divorcing family systems within a traditional psychoeducation group setting creates discomfort, and complex emotions and dysregulation result as the child recalls potentially painful memories and has limited resources for management of the overall system. However, the intervention manual we propose uses movement and breath work in the form of yoga to target lower brain stem activation and soothe a distressed physiology, dovetailing relational and educational material into an hour-long group session. Art and play are more suited for trauma interventions addressing adverse life experience. They create opportunity for the body to relax through metaphor within the response and facilitate children's verbal reports of emotionally laden events by reducing anxiety, thus helping the child to access memories and organize narratives (Malchiodi 2012). Each session ends with cognitive processing; however, this is delivered through the lens of play and art to provide a developmentally appropriate means of communicating and retains a whole brain process to reduce stress.

Rationale for using animal narratives in the curriculum

The curriculum below includes animals as a predominant theme. We incorporate the therapy dogs at our clinic (who quickly have become celebrities of sorts) for the children participating in these groups. Children are naturally drawn to animals and have connected their story outlined in each curriculum with the animal character, including their personalities, family system and somatic experience. We have modified our curricula over time to include children's perspectives, and continue to refine the stories of these dogs to incorporate the wisdom provided by children. Our goal was to identify the multi-faceted nature of these adverse experiences and the nuances of a child's worldview. Similar to concepts within the family yoga interview, therapy dogs are brought into group session at the end for the cognitive processing portion of the group for a conversational process session. The children can ask questions or, more often, provide examples of their own story including how it is similar or different from the dog's. They relate to one another in this process and this portion of the group session offers an opportunity for us to better understand the child's process in order to dovetail psychoeducation or normalization of experience as needed. Live animals can be replaced by puppets or other prop-based interventions for those who are not involved in animal assisted human health but want to have similar experiential work.

Yoga and play to facilitate the group process

It is important to note that the curricula we created for group work are different than what you may experience in yoga practice outside of a clinical setting. Typically, in yoga group work at a studio, there is a relaxing flow to the yoga sequencing or clear ordering of the yoga poses based on the theme of the day and how the facilitator may want to incorporate other limbs of yoga practice into their teaching. The stories we created are designed to convey psychoeducation and normalize lived experience and will often feel a little clunky for yoga professionals. We purposefully shifted the sequencing for kids engaged in these groups to retain their attention, after many group sessions of trial and error of yoga sequencing within the narratives. The narratives below are the basic story and the therapist will elaborate and/or draw upon repetition within the story to shift movement from the right side of the body to stretch or balance with the left side of the body. Children may interject ideas into the story and our recommendation is to utilize a child-centered perspective, incorporating whenever possible the group members' ideas or experiences into the narrative. This yoga style is grounded in the practice of *Imagination Yoga*, which includes the facilitator being encouraged to ask children to describe the room, if the story is painting a scene, describe their object or describe characteristics of the yoga pose to bring the story to life. An example of this would be a story about a crown being pulled from a treasure chest (forward bend to reach towards a treasure chest, grab the crown and move into staff pose, lifting your hands high above your head to place the crown on top of your head). The facilitator may stop and describe the crown, the style and color of jewels and open the room up to children offering descriptions of their own crowns. The inclusive imaginative process within yoga narratives will also provide assessment data or insight into a child's perspective, self-worth, family system or experience. The goal is for children to achieve focus and remain regulated throughout the session as they absorb the content and process of the work. The yoga narratives are designed to last approximately 15–20 minutes during a one-hour group.

Play therapy and expressive arts are incorporated into the curriculum following the yoga narrative. This is to allow creative expression and further processing and integration of content. The play and expressive art content will also provide the child with an opportunity to "make it their own," shifting into the child's process, drawing upon metaphor within the application. The process is relational through the group interaction with children working together to problem solve and engage in the play therapy game or art activity, aligning with the theme or content from the yoga narrative. The play therapy or expressive art activity typically is 20–30 minutes in length during the one-hour group. This allows for 10–15 minutes of processing for cognitive engagement and involvement of AAIs or puppet work if integrating this modality.

The group sequence ends with cognitive processing through group facilitation. Again, this is where the group curriculum below incorporates animal assisted human health through a therapy animal brought into session. We do not have our therapy dogs in the group throughout the process, as incorporating the animal during yoga can create disruption with flow. Children can become distracted when the handler is providing feedback, regulation and direction to their animal partner, as coming into a room full of children is exciting for a dog! However, bringing the animal into the last 10–15 minutes of the group provides just the right amount of time and interaction for the goals of the group curriculum and process.

Directive children's divorce support group narrative: examples for initial sessions

WEEK 1: "THE NEW PUP IN TOWN"
Goals

1. To assist in introductions and beginning conversations around connection with others and the idea of divorce occurring in a family system.

2. To build relationships and therapeutic rapport.

3. To investigate strengths; naming and experiencing inherent strengths of the child.

4. To provide introduction to the mind and body, beginning awareness of the nervous system through narratives.

5. To provide introduction to yoga and movement, building confidence with yoga movement.

Materials

1. Yoga mats

2. Narrative "The New Pup in Town"

3. Sensor stick

4. Capes

5. Paint, brushes, markers and/or fabric pens

6. Drop cloth (optional)

7. Hula hoop

"The New Pup in Town" yoga narrative

Take three full yoga breaths. Put one hand on the floor and reach up to the sky **(side stretch)**. Look up and take a deep breath (repeat for both sides).

Olive the dog goes to the park after puppy school on Friday. She's a new pup in town. Her parents are divorcing, and she has moved to a different house with her mom. Olive is about to start her new school on Monday and feels SO nervous. Her body feels tight where she breathes and sometimes she has sweaty paws and it feels like ants are in her pants. She looks around the park and sees two dogs, Chloe and Apollo, playing together.

Olive is alone, sniffing trees, and looks up, up, up to the top of the tree **(tree pose)**, the branches sway in the breeze and she takes a few stretches which calm her nerves **(full body stretch)**. The nervous feelings seem to be moving out, but her body needs more stretching **(downward dog moves into cow and cat)**.

Olive notices in her body she is lonely, watching Chloe and Apollo play. Olive musters up the courage **(big full yoga breath)** to go over, and asks to play. Chloe and Apollo are happy to include her – how kind! Chloe, Apollo and Olive romp through the park, and Olive notices that when she isn't so nervous she can think and pretend with her imagination! They pretend to be dinosaurs **(Warrior 1/letting out big growls)**, astronauts soaring through space **(rocket ship... 321 blastoff)** and fish swimming through the ocean **(bow pose)**.

Olive and Chloe's moms trade numbers and decide to schedule a playdate that weekend. On Monday Apollo walks to school with Chloe and learns about the playdate which didn't include him. Apollo feels left out **(child's pose/sadness)**. Apollo decides to play with a different group at recess, but he doesn't have as much fun and wonders about his sad feelings. He misses Chloe, but also has a double dip feeling of being angry at her **(volcano pose...about to erupt)** for leaving him out. Apollo takes a breath and thinks, thinks, thinks **(downward dog)**. This is confusing, but he decides to talk to Chloe. He has hurt feelings.

(Namaste pose). At school, Chloe notices Apollo hasn't played with her since two recesses ago! She is confused and worried **(big full yoga breath)** and goes to ask Apollo if they're still friends. Apollo says yes, but his feelings were confused and hurt by Chloe's playing with Olive without him. Chloe didn't realize he felt left out and reassures Apollo they can all be friends. Apollo notices his body feels better **(full body stretch)**. Chloe invites both Apollo and Olive over for a playdate. All three play outside next to the creek **(Saturn/tight-rope walker)**, chase butterflies **(butterfly pose)**, eat treats and relax in their dog beds **(relaxation pose)** at Chloe's house. Apollo and Chloe feel better, and Olive is happy, realizing she has made two new friends. She has a new house; her family is changing but she also has two friends during this hard time in her life.

(Bringing the group back to a **Namaste pose**.)

Olive found out she has the superpower of making friends! Chloe has the superpower of courage! Apollo discovered he has the superpower of talking it through and keeping his cool!

(Move into expressive art and play activity "What's Your Super-power?")

Expressive art and play: "Capturing our Superpowers through Creative Capes"

Facilitator information: This activity is designed to help kids begin to think about strengths. Therapists can draw upon the theoretical framework of a strengths-based perspective to help assist children in developing ideas about what characteristics or abilities stand out as a means of coping with adverse experiences. Therapists can utilize the example processing questions or facilitate using their own words.

Bridging linguistic processing with an expressive art creates the opportunity for a whole brain activity. Provide the children with art materials that will be sufficient for working on a fabric cape. Images, pictures, words or any symbol can be utilized to represent the strengths or "superpower" a child has identified. These are their strengths or gifts they bring to their body, mind or the world. Deepen the experience by helping children identify something about how the power works; for example, "I have the power of courage!" (therapist deepening awareness) or "I can try new things even when I feel a little nervous."

Once the cape is created, use the hula hoop as "center stage" for children to name their superpower. Strike the "superhero" pose when in the center of the hoop, boldly announcing your strength; for example, "I have the power of courage! I try new things even when I'm a little nervous."

[*Modification for family systems*: Have each member of the family create their cape and process utilizing family systems intervention. Utilize the hula hoop for individuals within the family to boldly name their power. Discuss roles and abilities of family members and how the family comes together to create one central system. All superpowers combine to create a super family! If needed you can "expand your hula hoop" through creating a larger circle (we use pool noodles to create a larger oval or masking tape on the floor) or you can have your family members get close in one hula hoop to shout out their family powers.]

Reinforce children's strengths and declarations verbally. Children can march in a slow and steady rhythmic pacing, repeating their strength for neural integration (EMDR installation of a positive cognition).

End the session through the playful use of a sensor stick.

Narration for the group process: "We all have superpowers; the electricity and power in our body provides us the ability to do amazing things. You can see this power through the sensor stick by using your hands to complete the circuit."

Have kids complete the circuit with the sensor stick (warning, this usually gets giggly and silly!). Create further connection with the group [or family system] by using one sensor stick to complete a group human circuit and process the power of community, friendship and connection with other kids [or family members].

[Animal partner and handler enter for therapeutic support during processing questions if using animal assisted interventions.]

Example processing questions

1. Olive has just moved because her parents are divorced. She said she was nervous, but what other kinds of feelings could she be having?

2. For some, making friends can be hard when you are feeling new and for others it seems easy. What do you think?

3. Talent and superpowers can be discovered! Superpowers are who we are or what we bring to our body, mind or to the world. What is a superpower you have? What is something about you that makes you feel strong or powerful?

WEEK 2: "CALM AND STORMY TIMES"
Goals

1. To assist in beginning conversations of how divorce can impact our body and mind.

2. To introduce neurobiology and concepts of the brain and nervous system.

3. To investigate regulation and how we bring our body back into an "all is well" space.

4. To use yoga and play, building confidence with yoga movement and expressive arts for conversations about coping skills.

Materials

1. Yoga mats

2. Narrative "Calm and Stormy Times"

3. Blank or non-printed umbrellas

4. Paint, brushes, markers and/or fabric pens

5. Drop cloth (optional)

6. Puff balls, feathers

7. Thunder tube (optional)

"Calm and Stormy Times" yoga narrative

Take three full yoga breaths. Put one hand on the floor and reach up to the sky **(side stretch)**. Look up and take a deep breath (repeat for both sides).

Sometimes our body needs help to get back to where we feel calm and have a feeling that all is well. Today, let's hear about what happened when Olive first heard about her parents getting divorced **(hero pose)**. Be sure to pay attention to your body! Our breath and mind (point to chest/lungs and brain) are the key to not getting lost or overwhelmed by a feelings storm. Let's go!

Olive was getting ready to eat dinner **(chair pose)** as her mom fixed her favorite meal, dog bones over peanut butter. Olive's mom sat down **(chair pose)** and asked if Olive had noticed that her mom and dad would often growl and bark loudly at each other. Olive nodded (like all the time she thought). Olive's mom explained that sometimes moms and dads don't get along anymore and decide to get divorced **(staff pose)**. When Olive heard this, she felt like she was sinking, sinking, sinking **(forward bend)** into the floor. It seemed like she had sunk into a vast ocean and was on a boat all alone in the middle of a great big water **(boat pose)**. She looked down to see two oars. She picked up one oar in each paw and looked up. Above her head were dark clouds and the first drip drop of rain began to fall on her head. Olive thought, I am so MAD! Row, Row, Row the Boat. MAD MAD! Row, Row, Row the Boat. MAD MAD MAD! The rain is really falling now and the wind is picking up fast! Wow! Olive, watch out those are some BIG waves! Row, Row, Row the Boat. Row, Row, Row the Boat. Row, Row, Row the Boat. Stop. Pause, legs down, BIG WAVE…**(forward bend)**. SPLASH! Body scan. My heart is beating faster, *the breath inside my body* is rapid (very fast) and I am having short breaths, not like a big star breath at all **(staff pose)**.

My SYMPATHETIC nervous system is turned on. This happens when our bodies are big with the feeling of a fight or flight, like when we're mad or scared or worried! We need to use our superpower yoga breath to help Olive and our bodies too. YOGA STAR BREATH in and out, but the out is a *super out* or longer than the in **(repeat breath work as many times as needed)**. Stop. Pause. Body scan. My heart is beating slower, the *breath inside my body* is slow and steady. Yes! We did it! Our PARASYMPATHETIC nervous system is in balance once again. This happens when you get back into your "all is well place." No more Mad. We helped Olive!

The clouds are now behind Olive and she can see rays of sun and a shoreline. She wonders if her family will be happier divorced.

Less barking and growling. Olive gets ready to paddle to the shore. Gha! One of her paddles is missing thanks to that storm back there. She thinks "I can get frustrated and mad about this or do something about it." Problem solving skills are easier when you have your superpower PARASYMPATHETIC nervous system in balance. Breathe in and out with the super out longer than your in. We can think better in our "all is well" place. Yes! Eureka! She can use one paddle and her boat is now a kayak **(boat pose…kayak style)**. Great. We're safely paddling to shore.

Let's get out of our boats and gaze upon this new land. Olive realizes her family is changing…maybe it won't be so bad. Birds seem to be dancing in the sky **(airplane pose)**. Olive can dance too! **(dancer pose)**. Up ahead is a large mountain **(mountain pose)**. We are at rest…all is well… Olive's mom explains that they will be selling the house and that she and her mom will be moving to an apartment, which means she will have to go to a new school. Olive feels like the ground under her mountain is starting to rumble, rumble, rumble (feet movement in place/running in place). The mountain up ahead **(mountain pose)** is beginning to look more and more like a volcano! Olive is MAD. Steam is releasing from the top in big, BIG, BIGGER bursts **(volcano pose, movement in hands moves up the body to an exploding point)**. The volcano is erupting! BARK BARK BARK… HOWLLLLLL! **(sequences of volcano pose)**. Stop. Pause. Body scan **(resting mountain pose move into downward dog)**. Olive notices the MAD and her SYMPATHETIC nervous system has her heart beating fast, and she also notices how her heart is beating fast. Olive's brain is thinking, thinking, thinking… How does she get her brain back? Olive takes in her big yoga breath with a super out longer than her in **(breath)**. She now can think things through **(hero pose)**.

Olive imagines her new apartment being at the top of a tower in a beautiful forest. Her room would be painted in gold glitter sparkles. At the base of the biggest tree is a big frog **(frog pose)**. As she looks up, up, up towards the branches **(tree pose)** she can see the sky slowly changing to nightfall with stars up above. The branches sway gently from side to side. Up ahead is a big harvest moon **(moon pose)**. Olive feels tired from all her big stormy feelings.

She notices a peaceful empty cave waiting just for her. She moves into the cave **(child's pose)** and checks in with her body. Olive is warm and stretches out on her back **(savasana/relaxation pose)**. Yes, all is well tonight and she lies in her bed for sleep.

Move into expressive art and play activity "Staying Dry in a Feelings Storm" adapted from Paris Goodyear-Brown's "Coping Umbrellas" (Goodyear-Brown 2010).

Narrative and artful play

We experienced both our sympathetic nervous system and parasympathetic nervous system today as we heard about when Olive discovered her parents getting a divorce. One part of the story had us in a feelings storm with rain and wind. The ways in which we cope during times of stress are how we help our body stay calm. Today we're going to end our time together talking about all the different ways we can help our body and minds find an "all is well" calm place. This could be through DOING things or BEING things (moving our bodies or changing our environments are doing things; telling our brains helpful words or focusing on our surroundings in mindfulness are being things). Everyone is different! We are all different and what helps my body may or may not help your body stay calm. Sometimes we need to be a scientist and try new things to see what works. We're going to think about eight different things we can do to help stay calm during a feelings storm. Then we're going to paint or draw these skills on an umbrella as a reminder for how to stay dry during the next feelings storm that comes our way.

"Staying Dry in a Feelings Storm" with our umbrella: a reminder of all the ways we can calm our body

We are going to write words or use pictures to represent our strategies for staying calm during a feelings storm. Remember these can be doing things or being things that help us keep our body calm and protected.

After creating the expressive art tool with representations of all the various coping skills you can use a playful expression of the skill by having kids practice their breathing, say their words of affirmation as you stand on a stool and toss cotton balls or other soft toys into the sky and experience them bouncing off the umbrella and away from the body. All is well. **Namaste**.

Process the various coping skills or different approaches kids thought of to calm their body through group conversation. This can incorporate AAIs or puppets.

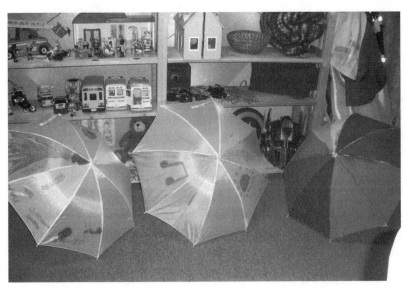

Figure 4.1 Example of group work creating coping umbrellas

Creating directive curriculum for addressing specific adverse experiences, such as divorce, will build upon the previous week's learning. Concepts introduced early on will be reviewed in later weeks to solidify children's learning or their understanding of material. Learning occurs best within a social environment, reinforced by Carl Rogers in his writings on education and curriculum. Rogers (1961) emphasized that experiential learning within a social environment provides a personally meaningful practice, having a quality of emotion in conjunction with the cognitive process to create successful outcomes. A group process that has a focus on both education and processing of complex material needs a foundation of safety to ensure the group can move through content, while balancing the benefits of group with the ethical considerations of multi-person processes.

Benefits and ethical considerations of group and family therapy

There are multiple benefits in incorporating yoga movement and play into family systems or group work. First, we often hear concerns about space and/or materials needed for becoming successful in this practice. Many therapists can feel overwhelmed by costs associated with additional training (most of us are still trying to pay off our student loans from graduate studies!) and the sheer number of materials needed to practice, including a wide variety of miniatures, art supplies, puppet selections, toys, books, etc. A very basic deck of yoga picture cards can be created by a crafty therapist using even a simple photography application on a cell phone and support from a willing family member or friend to photograph yoga poses. These can be printed at low cost and laminated to withstand multiple uses. Otherwise, there are many yoga cards on the market with drawings and explanations of poses that can be purchased at a reasonable price. To utilize directive yoga narratives, as outlined in the first two sessions of the divorce group curriculum, materials can be purchased inexpensively, or the play and art-based intervention can be modified to incorporate even more basic materials that can be found within the school supply section of a store. The limited number of materials also means the process becomes highly mobile and accessible for school-based therapists, hospital-based counseling or child life specialists. Yoga and play are versatile for individual or family therapy sessions in community-based practice settings for counselors and family skill builders who travel from home to home with their equipment.

There are ethical considerations for this work, including having knowledge of family systems, child development, trauma and trauma-informed therapeutic interventions, animal assisted human health (if incorporating a therapy animal), play therapy practices and training in yoga to safely and successfully integrate these concepts or interventions. We recommend training and/or a certification program to ensure adequate professional education benchmarks have been met, prior to incorporating this type of work into practice; there are some very affordable options available. We also encourage ongoing supervision and peer consultation for feedback and support throughout a career. This creates an ability to continue to develop ideas, ask for support for vicarious traumatization and find clarity for cases which bring puzzlement or the therapist having the feeling of being stuck. It is important to have adequate training for malpractice insurance purposes as this will provide support to your work if ever a complaint is issued to a licensing board regarding your clinical practice. Additionally, many of us who work in a trauma field are called to testify in court related to family custody matters, abuse, trauma or criminal proceedings and need to be able to clearly articulate not only our training but depth of knowledge, while providing testimony to support the work and successfully advocate for the child.

CHAPTER 5

Concluding Thoughts

SELF-CARE AND FUTURE RESEARCH

Remembering and building upon past knowledge

Judith Herman (1992) emphasized that, in our profession of mental health, we have understood trauma in the past and over time it has been discovered and lost repeatedly across centuries. The aspects of care for those who are impacted by adversity continue to move on a pendulum swing of remembering and forgetting. What is creating the phenomenon of our inability to remember and build upon the past? Our goal in this text includes taking a close look at the field's rich research history, foundational concepts of play therapy, biology, art, animal assisted human health and yoga to integrate and build a model which honors the work done earlier. We hope clinicians and researchers are not missing looking toward the past to strengthen and build upon existing work as they seek to discover something new for the future. We stand on the shoulders of giants; let's continue to build a way of engagement, intervention and assessment of outcomes that is inclusive rather than exclusive.

Advancement in education and training

The model of engagement described in this text is one which requires us to move beyond the basics and specialize within our practice. The components necessary for autocatalytic outcomes, and to approach a case incorporating a mind–body connection, require basic education and clinical training in mental health theory, child development and diagnostics, but also require advanced coursework and education in pediatric trauma and expressive arts. There are numerous legal and ethical components when counseling children. Popular graduate school textbooks training clinicians to work with individuals, groups and families often mention ethical issues related to treating pediatric populations only briefly, primarily focusing on confidentiality and abuse reporting laws (Sori and Hecker 2015). However, child trauma treatment is a specialty and carries with it many ethical considerations. Ethical involvement of play, touch, movement, art, animals, record-keeping and complexities with divorcing family systems, including parental rights versus custody arrangements, are just a few considerations therapists juggle when developing treatment plans and facilitating care. Comprehensive education and support are paramount for therapists to feel knowledgeable, professionally safe and successful within their work.

We understand that training and advanced knowledge in the areas of play therapy, trauma theory, neurobiology and animal assisted human health (if incorporating) are necessary to ethically incorporate the practice successfully. There are a multitude of training options available; however, we urge caution during selection. Scrutiny of presenter or instructor history, education and training level, along with learning objectives and whether the training will align with your long-term goals, is important when selecting a workshop or program. Clinicians seeking to advance their knowledge of play therapy or gain certification as a registered play therapist will want to ensure play therapy trainings are approved by the Association for Play Therapy and the facilitator is an approved provider for Play Therapy Education. This designation will safeguard your training by the trainer meeting criteria and guidelines for becoming a registered play therapist as well as meeting standards outlined by experts in the field.

There are limited accreditation processes for coursework and certification programs post-graduate. There may not always be a governing board which oversees educational certification programs. Specific criteria or standards seen in accredited graduate education programs for psychology, social work, counseling or other related disciplines have boards which govern their competencies and student learning outcomes. Post-graduate education certification programs need therapist evaluation to determine whether they are reputable and will provide the education required for advancing your career. An instructor or facilitator who has education, but does not practice in the field, manage a caseload or navigate the complexities of how their book knowledge may translate into clinical practice, often lacks perspective. Alternatively, an instructor or set of facilitators who have ample practice-based experience, but have never advanced their education beyond the basics of graduate school, may lack specialized and supervised training to successfully understand applications of specialty programs within clinical practice. Training programs which support continuing education should be approved by licensing boards for continuing education credits. This can be an expensive process, which is a deterrent for many instructors who want to drive down the cost of workshops for participants. However, this approval does require a peer review of the course abstract and learning objectives, along with the facilitator's policy for business practice. This process offers the workshop attendee some peace of mind that there have been checks and balances associated with creating course content.

Educators, facilitators or instructors should be able to provide you feedback about their own training and education process, including supervision for implementing interventions. The designation of "RPT" or "RPT-S" indicates a registered play therapist or registered play therapy supervisor and can be a positive sign that your facilitator has received advanced training and supervision in the field of play therapy. Animal assisted human health programs should have, at a minimum, a curriculum which provides comprehensive training for ethics, including animal welfare ethics and malpractice considerations. Education on animal behavior, applications to mental health practice and standards for mitigating health risks, thereby reducing zoonotic concerns in a health care practice, should all be components of animal assisted training programs.

The cost of caring: burnout

We have discussed in this text how larger systems can add pressure onto a therapist in the fee-for-service model. Agencies or private practice settings have a focus on the bottom line because the need for revenue impacts the ability to continue providing support. Insurance companies seek to drive down the reimbursement costs to therapists of direct payment for care, seeing record-breaking profits because of the strategy in the United States. To offset the lower wage, therapists try to find ways to squeeze more clients into an already full caseload in an attempt at recovering some of the financial loss. This ensures they can keep the lights on and continue doing the work that they spent a decade or more learning how to do well. Any system which cannot support those who support the suffering creates a steady state of burnout.

The level of empathy, care, compassion and dedication to pursue helping those who suffer carries with it a higher probability of burnout. The process of burnout is described by Maslach (1982) as a psychological syndrome in response to chronic interpersonal stressors on the job cumulatively contributing to the individual or population served by an organization. This is a meta-construct with three distinct factions: emotional exhaustion, depersonalization and reduced sense of personal accomplishment (Maslach 1982, 1998). Burnout, once a steady state of emotional exhaustion has set in, develops a sensation of having nothing left to give. Consequently, as a result of burnout, therapists may pigeonhole people into various categories and then respond to that stereotype or category rather than seeing the person as an individual adapting to adversity within their life. It is common in this field to hear people speak of their clients by the diagnosis assigned as explanation for the exasperation felt. It is common to hear clients referred to as "frequent fliers" or "over-utilizers" when they struggle with finding reprieve from their mental health symptoms. This is a form of depersonalization and a process of burnout. Looking at people in the worst possible light rather than finding their strengths is a symptom low of energy and ambition because of burnout. Therefore, it is also common to hear us in the field talk about a person's coping skills negatively as they struggle with addiction, disordered eating or self-harming behavior. This negative conversation is often a sign that the therapist needs detachment. Detaching emotionally creates a buffer between therapist and client and is a call for help by clinicians either needing a change or more support from their community.

Burnout drives us towards a practice where we "show up" but are not actually present with our clients. I remember some years ago, during long weeks and months of double shifts every day and the weekend work required for building the mental health clinic, finding I was in a space of feeling burned out. This was captured by a six-year-old client I was working with who, during a session, stopped her play in the sandtray to tap me on the forehead with her index finger: "Are you there miss Michelle?" What a wake-up call! She was correct; in that moment I wasn't there as my mind had drifted to the worries associated with surviving managed care changes. She brought me back to the present and highlighted the importance of taking care of myself, knowing when to ask for help and support so that I, in turn, could support her as she engaged in therapy.

Anyone can experience burnout within a job setting or career; however, human service professionals have the added accompanying phenomenon of compassion fatigue. Caring people can experience the pain and suffering of others as a direct result of engagement within the work.

The cost of caring: compassion fatigue

Secondary traumatic stress or compassion fatigue as described by Figley (1995) covers the process of secondary stress when helping or wanting to help a suffering person. We discuss within this text the need for exquisite empathy and deep attunement for the therapist to enter a room, both in a state of vulnerability and readiness to experience the child's world. This inherently includes suffering, as we specialize in helping those who face adverse experiences and trauma.

The nature of working within mental health settings requires us to look at problems. We begin with assessment, often by focusing on problems. We ask about symptoms, behavioral issues, community factors impacting the child and family, and parents relate to us the situation in terms of deficits. This process usually involves tearful expressions of the problem with a plea for help or expectation that we will fix it. Parents (and managed care) want rapid results or have expectations we will be in a different place in a few short weeks. The focus on problems often drives out time or opportunity to look for strengths and find hope. The focus on problems, coupled with anxiety and added stress for rapid change, can result in our inability to appreciate the process.

Therapy is an evolution; very infrequently do we have one groundbreaking insight or connection after another as each session unfolds. Typically, children will come into treatment and we will experience repetition within the play or walk away with very little new information from the week before. The repetition could be indicative of the trauma or a child immersed within post-traumatic play as they sequentially integrate their experience. The sessions may carry one small piece of information each week that, after some time, when all put together, reveal a larger theme or issue. The therapy processing as an evolution is also a part of the autocatalytic process we have described throughout this book. We find it unrealistic to assume a therapist will find the exact theory-based intervention or combination of theories in an integrated fashion correctly the first time. We find that assessment of progress is ongoing as we modify our approach or tailor the ingredients of intervention to create change for a child. Thomas Edison is famous for discussing having not failed 10,000 times or failing even once while creating a lightbulb. Instead, Edison discusses eliminating the ways that will not work to find ways that will work and become successful (Woodside 2009). We have sessions that are slow, or interventions we walk away from thinking, "Well, that didn't go as planned" and regroup, analyze and get back to work finding ways that will create the change people are searching for. Therapy is an evolution; however, the pressure for fast results can create a sense of failure compounding compassion fatigue.

There is a focus on problems and we forget therapy is a slow evolution of change. Typically, what we will hear is therapists reflecting upon the lack of positive feedback. We all like to hear how well we are doing, but more often we hear about how well we are not doing, from parents who are speaking from a place of fear, anxiety, disbelief or frustration. High conflict divorce, child sexual abuse allegations, identification of domestic violence in the home, disclosure of physical punishment leaving bruises, parental mental health illness and school-based bullying are all typical issues of children experiencing adversity and all carry heavy emotion for parents. Therapists are often on the receiving end of that emotion and face criticism or negative feedback when a child is slow to improve or continues to engage in "behavior" at home. The lack of positive feedback or understanding of a process can contribute to an overall sense of compassion fatigue.

System stress

This work carries with it a high level of emotional stress. It requires a workplace system which can provide a balance for the therapist, so the system creates a holding space for the therapist to process the impact of the work. The system must assist in the ability for a therapist to intentionally enter a therapy session. Supervisors and colleagues help create a safe space to allow authentic expression of the impact this work leaves on our own physical and mental health. Healthy systems will have knowledge and understanding about the impact of caring for those who suffer and urge everyone to work together to create change. However, agencies or clinics face the struggle of burnout too, as they are embedded within the larger community environment, navigating demanding expectations related to policy structure, politics, development and finances. Therefore we all need time to reflect and understand the multiple perspectives or reasons behind system stress.

The input of every member of the system impacts the overall health of an organization. Chronic negativity, anger or blame towards individual members of the system or groups of people within the system (clients, administrators, clinicians) all contribute to a system's demise. Collective action can create change. Action needs to be on behalf of the therapist and staff who all contribute to system functioning. This can be reflected upon as a state of deep democracy. Democracy is often considered an ideal of a cohesive community of people working together in an effort towards finding fair solutions in a non-violent manner to reconcile conflict or solve problems (Bloom and Farragher 2013). This is not only a factor of behavior, but fundamental awareness to ensure there are checks and balances supporting a system. Deep democracy requires a change in awareness that all people contribute their ideas, points of view, energy or feelings to the system, changing it incrementally as they do (Bloom and Farragher 2013). This concept emphasizes the ecological fact of all being connected in a complex interdependent web. Burnout for one is contagious for another and will slowly impact the entire system. Everyone taking responsibility to support members of the system who are showing signs of burnout is critical for the system to move back into equilibrium or balance.

Countertransference and absorbing pain

Reflection on the work includes therapists looking closely at countertransference issues and what may be brought to the surface from their own history and narrative, while serving those with pasts which echo their own. Therapists who engage in this work are most successful when they can monitor their own physiology and emotions throughout the session and day, caring for their own needs, to regulate difficult sensory experiences as they come and having options for seeking support when needed. Bottling up the emotions associated with trauma work to "self-care" when you get home does not make sense. A relaxing bubble bath will not wash away all the day's stress that combined and compounded to create burnout and compassion fatigue. However, engagement within your own process to unpack what is impacting you throughout the day, taking time to regulate through conversation, your own art-making or movement means we practice what we teach our clients. Why can't we apply the principles of therapy to self-care during the day within and outside of sessions to ensure we leave the day with a greater sense of calm?

Maintaining strong compassion for yourself while navigating complex client cases and systems can be difficult, but is paramount as we explore the shared trauma response. Burnout can occur in any field. An accountant can feel and describe a sense of burnout;

however, an accountant will not describe experiencing a shared trauma experience and fatigue because of caring. We emphasize the need for not minimizing the phenomenon of experiencing workplace stress or the impact of working with trauma survivors.

Remembering who we are

Although it may feel at times that the work we do is hopeless, exhausting and we question a world where such harm can come to children, we can remind ourselves that we are not alone, and we are making an impact. There is a quote from Fred Rogers which captures who we are. Schulten (2017) reported it in her *New York Times* piece while reporting on Hurricane Harvey as she looked upon the pain, sorrow and impact of the storm. Fred Rogers stated, "When I was a boy and I would see scary things in the news, my mother would say to me, 'Look for the helpers. You will always find people who are helping.'" During times of disaster and times of sorrow, children and families look to us for support and guidance. We are the helpers and the work we are doing is helping change the life of a child, thus creating impact and change for the world.

Social and organizational change for support

One of the most difficult things to take on is large organizational or social change, as we talk about how to mitigate the effects of burnout and secondary traumatic stress. However, just as we may break down a large problem for clients seeking care into smaller, manageable pieces, could we not apply the construct to organizational change? Collective action through political advocacy could happen through professional groups or organizations. Membership of professional groups and organizations is a small way of enacting change and breaking down the problem. Once a therapist is a member, they then have representation for larger issues they want to have an impact on, and social change. Members on the inside of these organizations need on-the-ground workers to provide compelling human interest stories or to bring to life the issues that impact the clients they serve. Larger managed care issues of abuse of power and changing reimbursement rates are political and legislative issues that need a phone call, a letter or brief testimony of the problem. Membership of professional organizations that create collective action is one way to break down the problem and create social change.

Social change for the systems we live and work in also occurs through interdisciplinary work. Stepping outside of our own profession to talk with other professionals can create lasting change. Partnerships with other medical professionals working in primary care, specialty medical practices, occupational therapy, physical therapy and speech language pathology is a beginning. The work discussed in this text also crossed paths with education professionals, yoga professionals and veterinary doctors. We are all interconnected and often share common goals that we might not see until we begin the conversation. This type of collaboration breathes life back into the work, energizes us to be innovative and creates change for the larger systems as we develop new programs and advocate on shared interests.

Next steps for continued learning

There is much work to be done but let us not forget the past. Let us work together to continue to build upon research and history across professions to create more solidified interventions or new forms of clinical practice. The field of animal assisted human health is still young and developing. We need more clinicians who are interested in the work and have the ambition to record their cases in meaningful ways to contribute to the field. Play therapy is infinite in creativity and further exploration will continue to refine and broadcast to the world of academia and other professions what children need within mental health counseling. Continued work and research will continue to further the field of medical neuroscience and trauma. All of us are needed in advancing this work, as technology and understanding grows, connecting the knowledge of the past with the future.

We are the helpers during times of sorrow, terror or despair. May we not forget our importance in the life of a child and the change that we subsequently bring to the world. As we reflect on the interconnected web of disciplines impacting our work, theories, intervention styles, individual personality and limitless opportunities for creative expression, may we also find room for honoring that we call our work a *practice*. Let every day be a day we can forgive a setback, find kindness for another and contribute even in a small way to advocacy and change. Let every day be a day we can practice with the knowledge that we are enough.

References

Abramowitz, C.V. (1976) The effectiveness of group psychotherapy with children. *Archives of General Psychiatry 33,* 320–326.

Abrams, S. (2001) Summation-unrealized possibilities: Comments on Anna Freud's normality and pathology in childhood. *Psychoanalytic Study of the Child 56,* 105–119.

Aiello, S.E. (2016) *The Merck Veterinary Manual,* 11th edn. Kenilworth, NJ: Merck.

Almon, J.W. (2017) Restoring play: The march goes on. In M.R. Moore and C. Sabo-Risley (eds) *Play in American Life.* Bloomingdale, IN: Archway Publishing.

American Art Therapy Association (2013) *What Is Art Therapy?* Alexandria, VA: American Art Therapy Association.

American Psychiatric Association (2013) *Diagnostic and Statistical Manual of Mental Disorders,* 5th edn. Arlington, VA: American Psychiatric Association.

American Psychological Presidential Task Force (May–June 2006) Evidence-based practice in psychology. *American Psychologist 61,* 4, 271–285.

Anda, R.F., Felitti, V.J., Bremner, D., Walker, J.D. *et al.* (2006) The enduring effects of abuse and related adverse experiences in childhood: A convergence of evidence from neurobiology and epidemiology. *European Archives of Psychiatry and Clinical Neuroscience 256,* 174–186.

Andersen, S.L. and Teicher, M.H. (2004) Stress, sensitive periods and maturational events in adolescent depression. *Trends in Neurosciences 33,* 4, 183–191.

Anderson, S.M. and Gedo, P.M. (2013) Relational trauma: Using play therapy to treat a disrupted attachment. *The Menninger Foundation 77,* 3, 250–268.

Applegate, J.S. and Shapiro, J.R. (2005) *Neurobiology for Clinical Social Work: Theory and Practice.* New York: Norton.

Arvidson, J., Kinniburgh, K., Howard, K., Evans, M. *et al.* (2011) Treatment of complex trauma in young children: Developmental and cultural considerations in application of the ARC intervention model. *Journal of Child & Adolescent Trauma 4,* 34–51.

Axline, V.A. (1969) *Play Therapy.* New York: Ballantine.

Badenoch, B. (2008) *Being a Brain-Wise Therapist: A Practical Guide to Interpersonal Neurobiology.* New York: Norton.

Badenoch, B. (2018) *The Heart of Trauma.* New York: Norton.

Beeferman, D. and Orvaschel, H. (1994) Group psychotherapy for depressed adolescents: A critical review. *International Journal of Group Psychotherapy 44,* 463–475.

Benedict, H.E. (2006) Object relations play therapy: Applications to attachment problems and relational trauma. In C.E. Schaefer and H.G. Kaduson (eds) *Contemporary Play Therapy.* New York: Guilford Press.

Berg, I.K. and Steiner, T. (2003) *Children's Solution Work.* New York: Norton.

Bergen, D. (2015) Psychological approaches to the study of play. *American Journal of Play 7,* 3, 101–128.

Berk, L.E. (2002) *Infants and Children: Prenatal through Middle Childhood.* Boston, MA: Allyn & Bacon.

Berzoff, J. (2016) *Inside Out and Outside In: Psychodynamic Clinical Theory and Psychopathology in Contemporary Multicultural Contexts.* Lanham, MD: Rowman & Littlefield.

Bloom, S.L. (2013) *Creating Sanctuary: Toward the Evolution of Sane Societies.* New York: Routledge.

Bloom, S.L. and Farragher, B. (2013) *Restoring Sanctuary: A New Operating System for Trauma-Informed Systems of Care.* New York: Oxford University Press.

Blumenfeld, H. (2018) *Neuroanatomy through Clinical Cases.* Oxford: Oxford University Press.

Booth, P.B. and Jernberg, A.M. (2009) *Theraplay: Helping Parents and Children Build Better Relationships through Attachment-Based Play.* New York: Wiley.

Bowlby, J. (1969) *Attachment and Loss: Volume I: Attachment.* London: Hogarth Press.

Bowlby, J. (1976) *Attachment and Loss: Volume II: Separation, Anger and Anxiety.* New York: Basic Books.

Briere, J. and Scott, C. (2006) *Principles of Trauma Therapy: A Guide to Symptoms, Evaluation and Treatment.* Thousand Oaks, CA: Sage.

Brown, B. (2010) *The Gifts of Imperfection: Let Go of Who You Think You're Supposed to Be and Embrace Who You Are: Your Guide to a Wholehearted Life.* Center City, MN: Hazelden Publishing.

Brown, K.W. and Cordon, S.L. (2009) Toward a phenomenology of mindfulness: Subjective experience and emotional correlates. In F. Didonna (ed.) *Clinical Handbook of Mindfulness.* New York: Springer.

Bury, R.G. (1961) *Plato Laws: English Translation.* Cambridge, MA: Harvard University Press.

Butler, K. (2013) *Therapy Dogs Today: Their Gifts, Our Obligation,* 2nd edn. Norman, OK: Funpuddle Publishing Associates.

Carey, S., Zaitchik, D. and Bascandziev, I. (2015) Theories of development: A dialog with Jean Piaget. *Developmental Review 38,* 36–54.

Carrion, V.G. and Wong, S.S. (2012) Can traumatic stress alter the brain? Understanding the implications of early trauma on brain development and learning. *Journal of Adolescent Health 51,* 523–528.

Carrion, V.G., Weems, C.F. and Reiss, A.L. (2007) Stress predicts brain changes in children: A pilot longitudinal study on youth stress, post-traumatic stress disorder and the hippocampus. *Pediatrics 119*, 3, 509–516.

Cassidy, J. (2008) The nature of a child's ties. In J. Cassidy and P.R. Shaver (eds) *Handbook of Attachment: Theory, Research and Clinical Applications*. New York: Guilford Press.

Cha, S. and Masho, S.W. (2014) Intimate partner violence and utilization of prenatal care in the United States. *Journal of Interpersonal Violence 29*, 5, 911–927.

Costin, L.B. (1997) *The Politics of Child Abuse in America*. Oxford: Oxford University Press.

Courtois, C.A. and Ford, J.D. (2013) *Treatment of Complex Trauma: A Sequenced, Relationship-Based Approach*. New York: Guilford Press.

Cronholm, P.F., Forke, C.M., Wade, R., Bair-Merritt, M.H. *et al.* (2015) Adverse childhood experiences: Expanding the concept of adversity. *American Journal of Preventive Medicine 49*, 3, 354–361.

Duhl, F.J., Kantor, D. and Duhl, B. (1973) Learning, space and action in family therapy: A primer of sculpture. In D.A. Bloch (ed.) *Techniques of Family Therapy: A Primer*. New York: Grune and Stratton.

Drewes, A.A. and Schaefer, C.E. (2014) Introduction: How play therapy causes therapeutic change. In C.E. Schaefer and A.A. Drewes (eds) *The Therapeutic Powers of Play: 20 Core Agents of Change*. Hoboken, NJ: Wiley.

Ener, L. (2016) The extraordinary beginning years: Birth to 2 years old. In D.C. Ray (ed.) *A Therapist's Guide to Child Development: The Extraordinarily Normal Years*. New York: Routledge.

Felitti, V.J., Anda, R.F., Nordenberg, D., Williamson, D.F. *et al.* (1998) Relationship of childhood abuse and household dysfunction to many of the leading causes of death in adults: The adverse childhood experiences (ACE) study. *American Journal of Preventive Medicine 14*, 4, 245–258.

Ferraro, A.J., Malespin, T., Oehme, K., Brunker, M. and Opel, A. (2016) Advancing co-parenting education: Toward a foundation for supporting positive post-divorce adjustment. *Child and Adolescent Social Work Journal 33*, 407–415.

Figley, C.R. (1995) Compassion fatigue: Toward a new understanding of the costs of caring. In B.H. Stamm (ed.) *Secondary Traumatic Stress: Self-Care Issues for Clinicians, Researchers and Educators*. Baltimore, MD: Sidran.

Findling, J.H., Bratton, S.C. and Henson, R.K. (2006) Development of the trauma play scale: An observation-based assessment of the impact of trauma on the play therapy behaviors of young children. *International Journal of Play Therapy 15*, 1, 7–36.

Fine, A.H. and Beck, A. (2010) Understanding our kinship with animals: Input for health care professionals interested in the human/animal bond. In A.H. Fine (ed.) *Handbook on Animal Assisted Therapy: Theoretical Foundations and Guidelines for Practice*, 3rd edn. Burlington, MA: Academic Press Elsevier.

Flach, C., Leese, M., Heron, J., Evans, J. *et al.* (2011) Antenatal domestic violence, maternal mental health and subsequent child behaviour: A cohort study. *International Journal of Obstetrics and Gynaecology*, 1383–1391.

Flanagan, L.M. (2016a) Object relations theory. In J. Berzoff, L.M. Flanagan and P. Hertz (eds) *Inside Out and Outside In: Psychodynamic Clinical Theory and Psychopathology in Contemporary Multicultural Contexts*, 4th edn. Lanham, MD: Rowman & Littlefield.

Follette, V.M. and Vijay, A. (2009) Mindfulness for trauma and posttraumatic stress disorder. In F. Didonna (ed.) *Clinical Handbook of Mindfulness*. New York: Springer.

Ford, J.D. and Cloitre, M. (2009) Best practices in psychotherapy for children and adolescents. In C.A. Courtois and J.D. Ford (eds) *Treating Complex Traumatic Stress Disorders*. New York: Guilford Press.

Fraley, R.C. and Heffernan, M.E. (2012) Attachment and parental divorce: A test of the diffusion and sensitive period. *Personality and Social Psychology Bulletin 39*, 9, 1199–1213.

Freud, S. (1896) Further remarks on the neuro-psychoses of defense. In *The Standard Edition of the Complete Psychodynamic Works of Sigmund Freud*. London: Hogarth Press.

Freud, S. (1963) *The Sexual Enlightenment of Children*. New York: Collier Books.

Freyd, J.J. (1996) *Betrayal Trauma: The Logic of Forgetting Childhood Abuse*. Cambridge, MA: Harvard University Press.

Friedmann, E., Son, H. and Tsai, C.C. (2010) The animal/human bond: Health and wellness. In A.H. Fine (ed.) *Handbook on Animal Assisted Therapy: Theoretical Foundations and Guidelines for Practice*, 3rd edn. Oxford: Elsevier.

Frost, J.L., Wortham, S.C. and Reifel, S.C. (2011) *Play and Child Development*, 4th edn. New York: Pearson.

Galantino, M.L., Galhavy, R. and Quinn, L. (2008) Therapeutic effects of yoga for children: A systematic review of the literature. *Pediatric Physical Therapy*, 66–80.

Galovan, A.M. and Schramm, D.G. (2017) Initial co-parenting patterns and post-divorce parent education programming: A latent class analysis. *Journal of Divorce and Remarriage 58*, 3, 212–226.

Gapp, K., Jawaid, A., Sarkies, P., Bohacek, J. *et al.* (2014) Implication of sperm RNAs in transgenerational inheritance of the effects of early trauma in mice. *Nature Neuroscience 17*, 5, 667–671.

Gaskill, R.L. and Perry, B.D. (2012) Child sexual abuse, traumatic experiences and their impact on the developing brain. In P. Goodyear-Brown (ed.) *Handbook of Child Sexual Abuse: Identification, Assessment and Treatment*. Hoboken, NJ: Wiley.

Gaskill, R.L. and Perry, B.D. (2014) The neurobiological power of play: Using the neurosequential model of therapeutics to guide play in the healing process. In C.A. Malchiodi and D.A. Crenshaw (eds) *Creative Arts and Play Therapy for Attachment Problems*. New York: Guilford Press.

Gesell, A. (1928) *Infancy and Human Growth*. New York: Macmillan.

Gibbons, K. (2015) *Integrating Art Therapy and Yoga Therapy: Yoga, Art and the Use of Intention*. London: Jessica Kingsley Publishers.

Gil, E. (1991) *The Healing Power of Play: Working with Abused Children*. New York: Guilford Press.

Gil, E. (2006) *Helping Abused and Traumatized Children: Integrating Directive and Nondirective Approaches*. New York: Guilford Press.

Gil, E. (2015) *Play in Family Therapy*, 2nd edn. New York: Guilford Press.

Gil, E. (2017) *Posttraumatic Play in Children: What Clinicians Need to Know*. New York: Guilford Press.

Ginsburg, K.R. (2007) The importance of play in promoting healthy child development and maintaining strong parent–child bonds. *American Academy of Pediatrics 119*, 1, 182–191.

Glover, V. (2016) Maternal stress during pregnancy and infant and child outcomes. In A. Wenzel (ed.) *The Oxford Handbook of Perinatal Psychology*. New York: Oxford University Press.

Goodall, J. and Bekoff, M. (2002) *The Ten Trusts: What We Must Do to Care for the Animals We Love*. San Francisco, CA: Harper.

Goodyear-Brown, P. (2010) *Play Therapy with Traumatized Children: A Prescriptive Approach*. Hoboken, NJ: Wiley.

Greenspan, S. (n.d.). 'Floortime: What is truly is, and what it isn't.' Retrieved from www.icdl.com/education/selfstudy/webradio/dirfloortimemodel

Grote-Garcia, S., Donaldson, T.F., Kajoina, O. and Clair, N.S. (2017) Social media as a 21st century playground. In M.R. Moore and C. Sabo-Risley (eds) *Play in American Life*. Bloomingdale, IN: Archway Publishing.

Harder, V.S., Mutiso, V.N., Khasakhala, L.I., Burke, H.M. and Ndetei, D.M. (2012) Multiple traumas, postelection violence and posttraumatic stress among impoverished Kenyan youth. *Journal of Traumatic Stress 25*, 64–70.

Harker, A. (2018) Social dysfunction: The effects of early trauma and adversity on socialization and brain development. In R. Gibb and B. Kolb (eds) *The Neurobiology of Brain and Behavioral Development*. San Diego, CA: Elsevier.

Havener, L., Gentes, L., Thaler, B., Megel, M.E., Baun, M.M. and Driscoll, F.A. (2001) The effects of a companion animal on distress in children undergoing dental procedures. *Issues in Comprehensive Pediatric Nursing 24*, 137–152.

Hayes, S.C., Strosahl, K.D. and Wilson, K.G. (2016) *Acceptance and Commitment Therapy: The Process and Practice of Mindful Change*, 2nd edn. New York: Guilford Press.

Henderson, D. and Thompson, C.L. (2015) *Counseling Children*, 9th edn. New York: Brooks Cole.

Herman, J.L. (1992) *Trauma and Recovery*. New York: Basic Books.

Hesse, E. (2008) The adult attachment interview: Protocol, method of analysis and empirical studies. In J. Cassidy and P.R. Shaver (eds) *Handbook of Attachment: Theory, Research, and Clinical Applications*, 2nd edn. New York: Guilford Press.

Hesse, E. and Main, M. (2000) *The Organized Categories of Infant, Child and Adult Attachment: Flexible vs. Inflexible Attention under Attachment-Related Stress*. Washington, DC: American Psychological Association.

Homeyer, L.E. and Sweeney, D.S. (2011) *Sandtray Therapy: A Practical Manual*, 2nd edn. New York: Routledge.

Hughes, V. (2014) Sperm RNA carries marks of trauma. *Nature 508*, 7496, 296–297.

Hunt, T.K.A., Slack, K.S. and Berger, L.M. (2016) Adverse childhood experiences and problems in middle childhood. *Child Abuse and Neglect, 67*, 391–402.

Irwin, E.C. and Malloy, E.S. (1975) Family puppet interview. *Family Process 14*, 179–191.

John, M. (2013) From Osler to the cone technique. *HSR Proceedings in Intensive Care and Cardiovascular Anesthesia 5*, 1, 57–58.

Johnson, J.L. (2015) The history of play therapy. In K. O'Conner (ed.) *Handbook of Play Therapy*. Hoboken, NJ: Wiley.

Kabat-Zinn, J. (1993) Mindfulness meditation: Health benefits of an ancient Buddhist practice. In D. Goleman and J. Gurin (eds) *Mind Body Medicine: How to Use Your Mind for Better Health*. Yonkers, NY: Consumer Reports Books.

Karr-Morse, R. and Wiley, M.S. (2012) *Scared Sick: The Role of Childhood Trauma in Adult Disease*. New York: Basic Books.

Katcher, A.H. and Beck, A.M. (2010) Newer and older perspectives on the therapeutic effects of animals and nature. In A.H. Fine (ed.) *Handbook on Animal-Assisted Therapy: Theoretical Foundations and Guidelines for Practice*, 3rd edn. Oxford: Elsevier.

Keshavan, M.S., Diwadkar, V.A., Debellis, M., Dick, E. *et al.* (2002) Development of the corpus callosum in childhood, adolescence and early adulthood. *Life Sciences 70*, 1909–1922.

Kestly, T. (2015) Sandtray and storytelling in play therapy. In D.A. Crenshaw and A.L. Stewart (eds) *Play Therapy: A Comprehensive Guide to Theory and Practice*. New York: Guilford Press.

Khalsa, S.B.S., Telles, S., Cohen, L. and McCall, T. (2016) Introduction to yoga in health care. In S.B.S. Khalsa, L. Cohen, T. McCall and S. Telles (eds) *The Principles and Practice of Yoga in Health Care*. Fountainhall: Handspring Publishing.

Klaff, D. (1988) *Sandplay*. Boston, MA: Sigo Press.

Klein, B.G. (2013) *Cunningham's Textbook of Veterinary Physiology*, 5th edn. St. Louis, MO: Elsevier.

Klein, M. (1955) *New Directions in Psycho-Analysis: The Significance of Infant Conflict in the Pattern of Adult Behaviour*. New York: Basic Books.

KPJR Films Production (Bob Edwards and Shannon Strione) (2015) *Paper Tigers* [DVD].

Kottman, T. (2001) *Play Therapy: Basics and Beyond*. Alexandria, VA: American Counseling Association.

Kruger, K.A. and Serpell, J.A. (2010) Animal-assisted interventions in mental health: Definitions and theoretical foundations. In A.H. Fine (ed.) *Handbook on Animal Assisted Therapy: Theoretical Foundations and Guidelines for Practice*, 3rd edn. Burlington, MA: Academic Press Elsevier.

Labonté, B., Suderman, M., Maussion, G., Navaro, L. *et al.* (2012) Genome-wide epigenetic regulation by early-life trauma. *Archive General Psychiatry 69*, 7, 722–731.

Landreth, G.L. (1991) *Play Therapy: The Art of the Relationship.* Muncie, IN: Accelerated Development Publishing.

Landreth, G.L. (2001) Facilitative dimensions of play in the play therapy process. In G.L. Landreth (ed.) *Innovations in Play Therapy: Issues, Process and Special Populations.* Philadelphia, PA: Brunner-Routledge.

Lebo, D. (1955) The development of play as a form of therapy: From Rousseau to Rogers. *American Journal of Psychiatry 112,* 418–422.

Lemmens, J.S., Valkenburg, P.M and Peter, J. (2011) Psychosocial causes and consequences of pathological gaming. *Computers in Human Behavior 27,* 144–152.

Levine, P.A. (1997) *Waking the Tiger: Healing Trauma.* Berkeley, CA: North Atlantic Books.

Levine, P.A. (2018) Polyvagal theory and trauma. In S.W. Porges and D. Dana (eds) *Clinical Applications of the Polyvagal Theory: The Emergence of Polyvagal-Informed Therapies.* New York: Norton.

Lillard, A.S. (2005) *Montessori: The Science behind the Genius.* Oxford: Oxford University Press.

Louv, R. (2008) *Last Child in the Woods: Saving Our Children from Nature-Deficit Disorder.* New York: Workmanship Publishing.

Lussier, A.A., Islam, S.A. and Kobor, M.S. (2018) Epigenetics and genetics of development. In R. Gibb and B. Kolb (eds) *The Neurobiology of Brain and Behavioral Development.* San Diego, CA: Elsevier.

Malchiodi, C.A. (1998) *Understanding Children's Drawings.* New York: Guilford Press.

Malchiodi, C.A. (2008) Creative interventions and childhood trauma. In C.A. Malchiodi (ed.) *Creative Interventions with Traumatized Children.* New York: Guilford Press.

Malchiodi, C.A. (2012) Art therapy and the brain. In C.A. Malchiodi (ed.) *Handbook of Art Therapy,* 2nd edn. New York: Guilford Press.

Maslach, C. (1982) Understanding burnout: Definitional issues in analyzing a complex phenomenon. In W.S. Paine (ed.) *Job Stress and Burnout.* Beverly Hills, CA: Sage.

Maslach, C. (1998) A multidimensional theory of burnout. In C.L. Cooper (ed.) *Theories of Organizational Stress.* Oxford: Oxford University Press.

McGoldrick, M. (1999) History, genograms, and the family life cycle: Freud in context. In B. Carter and M. McGoldrick (eds) *The Expanded Family Life Cycle: Individual Family and Social Perspectives,* 3rd edn. Boston, MA: Allyn & Bacon.

McGoldrick, M., Gerson, R. and Petry, S. (2008) *Genograms: Assessment and Intervention.* New York: Norton.

McNeil, C.B. and Hembree-Kigin, T.L. (2011) *Parent–Child Interaction Therapy,* 3rd edn. New York: Springer.

Meadows, S. (2018) *Understanding Child Development: Psychological Perspectives and Applications.* New York: Routledge.

Melson, G.F. (1988) Availability of and involvement with pets by children: Determinants and correlates. *Anthrozos 2,* 1, 45–52.

Melson, G.F. (2001) *Why the Wild Things Are: Animals in the Lives of Children.* Cambridge, MA: First Harvard University Press.

Mercer, J. (2006) *Understanding Attachment.* Westport, CT: Praeger.

Midgley, N. (2011) Test of time: Anna Freud's normality and pathology in childhood (1965). *Clinical Child Psychology and Psychiatry 16,* 3, 475–482.

Moore, D.S. (2015) *The Developing Genome: An Introduction to Behavioral Epigenetics.* New York: Oxford University Press.

Moore, K.L., Dalley, A.F. and Agur, A.M.R. (2014) *Clinically Oriented Anatomy.* Baltimore, MD: Lippincott, Williams & Wilkins.

Montessori, M. (2014) *The Montessori Method.* North Charleston, SC: CreateSpace.

Munns, E. (2011) Theraplay: Attachment-enhancing play therapy. In C. Schaefer (ed.) *Foundations of Play Therapy,* 2nd edn. New York: Wiley.

Newell, J.M. and MacNeil, G.A. (2010) Professional burnout, vicarious trauma, secondary traumatic stress and compassion fatigue: A review of theoretical terms, risk factors and preventive methods for clinicians and researchers. *Best Practices in Mental Health 6,* 2, 57–68.

Nolte, J. (2009) *The Human Brain: An Introduction to Its Functional Anatomy,* 6th edn. Philadelphia, PA: Mosby Elsevier.

Nugent, N.R., Goldberg, A. and Uddin, M. (2016) Topical review: The emerging field of epigenetics: Informing models of pediatric trauma and physical health. *Journal of Pediatric Psychology 41,* 1, 55–64.

Oaklander, V. (1988) *Windows to Our Children.* New York: Gestalt Journal Press.

O'Brien, J. and Smith, J. (2002) Childhood transformed? Risk perceptions and the decline of free play. *British Journal of Occupational Therapy 65,* 3, 123–128.

O'Connor, K. (2000) *The Play Therapy Primer.* Hoboken, NJ: Wiley.

Panksepp, J. and Biven, L. (2012) *The Archaeology of Mind: Neuroevolutionary Origins of Human Emotions.* New York: Norton.

Patterson, J., Williams, L., Edwards, T.M., Chamow, L. and Grauf-Grounds, C. (2009) *Essential Skills in Family Therapy: From the First Interview to Termination,* 2nd edn. New York: Guilford Press.

Pears, K. and Fisher, P.A. (2005) Neurodevelopmental, cognitive and neuropsychological functioning in preschool-aged foster children: Associations with prior maltreatment and placement history. *Developmental and Behavioural Pediatrics 2,* 112–122.

Peña, C.J., Monk, C. and Champagne, F.A. (2012) Epigenetic effects of prenatal stress on 11-hydroxysteroid dehydrogenase-2 in the placenta and fetal brain. *PLOS One 7,* 6, 1–9.

Perry, B.D. (2006) The neurosequential model of therapeutics: Applying the principles of neuroscience to clinical work with traumatized and maltreated children. In N.B. Webb (ed.) *Working with Traumatized Youth in Child Welfare.* New York: Guilford Press.

Pham, P. N., Vinck, P. and Stover, E. (2009) Returning home: Forced conscription, reintegration, and mental health status of former abductees of the Lord's Resistance Army in northern Uganda. *BMC Psychiatry 9,* 23, 1–24.

Polusny, M.A., Erbes, C.R., Thuras, P., Moran, A. *et al.* (2015) Mindfulness-based stress reduction for posttraumatic stress disorder among veterans. *Journal of American Medical Association 314*, 5, 456–465.

Porges, S.W. (2015) Making the world safe for our children: Down-regulating defense and upregulating social engagement to "optimize" the human experience. *Children Australia 40*, 114–123.

Porges, S.W. (2017) *The Pocket Guide to the Polyvagal Theory: The Transformative Power of Feeling Safe*. New York: Norton.

Presti, D.E. (2016) *Foundational Concepts in Neuroscience: A Brain-Mind Odyssey*. New York: Norton.

Purves, D., Augustine, G., Fitzpatrick, D., Hall, W.C., LaMantia, A.S. and White, L.E. (2012) *Neuroscience*, 5th edn. Sunderland, MA: Sinauer Associates.

Ramo-Fernandez, L., Schneider, A., Wilker, S. and Kolass, I. (2015) Epigenetic alterations associated with war trauma and childhood maltreatment. *Behavioral Sciences and the Law 33*, 701–721.

Ray, D.C. (2011) *Advanced Play Therapy: Essential Conditions, Knowledge, and Skills for Child Practice*. New York: Routledge.

Ray, D.C. (2016) An overview of child development. In D.C. Ray (ed.) *A Therapist's Guide to Child Development: The Extraordinarily Normal Years*. New York: Routledge.

Rogers, C. (1961) *On Becoming a Person: A Therapist's View of Psychotherapy*. Boston, MA: Houghton Mifflin.

Rousseau, J.J. (1979) *Emile on Education*. New York: Basic Books.

Rubin, J.A. (2005) *Child Art Therapy*. Hoboken, NJ: Wiley.

Sandman, C.A., Davis, E.P., Buss, C. and Glynn, L.M. (2012) Exposure to prenatal psychobiological stress exerts programming influences on the mother and her fetus. *Neuroendocrinology 95*, 8–21.

Sandman, C.A., Wadhwa, P.D., Chicz-DeMet, A., Dunkel-Schetter, C. and Porto, M. (1997) Maternal stress, HPA activity and fetal/infant outcome. *Annals of the New York Academy of Sciences 814*, 266–275.

Sapolsky, R.M. (1994) *Why Zebras Don't Get Ulcers: The Acclaimed Guide to Stress, Stress-Related Diseases, and Coping*, 3rd edn. New York: Holt.

Schaefer, C.E. (2011) *Foundations of Play Therapy*, 2nd edn. Hoboken, NJ: Wiley.

Schore, J.R. and Schore, A.N. (2008) Modern attachment theory: The central role of affect regulation in development and treatment. *Clinical Social Work Journal 36*, 9–20.

Schubach De Domenico, G. (1988) *Sand Tray World Play: A Comprehensive Guide to the Use of the Sand Tray in Psychotherapeutic and Transformational Settings*, 3 vols. Oakland, CA: De Domenico.

Schulten, K. (2017) Look for the helpers. *The New York Times*, August 30.

Shaffer, D.R. (1999) *Developmental Psychology: Childhood and Adolescence*, 5th edn. Pacific Grove, CA: Brooks Cole.

Shapiro, F. (2017) *Eye Movement Desensitization and Reprocessing (EMDR) Therapy: Basic Principles Protocols and Procedures*, 3rd edn. New York: Guilford Press.

Shapiro, S.L., Brown, K.W., Thorensen, C. and Plante, T.G. (2011) The moderation of mindfulness-based stress reduction effects by trait mindfulness: Results from a randomized controlled trial. *Journal of Clinical Psychology 67*, 3, 267–277.

Shelan, W. and Stewart, A.L. (2015) Attachment security as a framework in play therapy. In D.A. Crenshaw and A.L. Stewart (eds) *Play Therapy: A Comprehensive Guide to Theory and Practice.* New York: Guilford Press.

Shuffelton, A.B. (2012) Rousseau's imaginary friend: Childhood, play and suspicion of the imagination in Emile. *Educational Theory 62*, 3, 305–321.

Siegel, D.J. (2003) An interpersonal neurobiology of psychotherapy: The developing mind and the resolution of trauma. In M.F. Solomon and D.J. Siegel (eds) *Healing Trauma: Attachment, Mind, Body, and Brain.* New York: Norton.

Siegel, D.J. (2012) *The Developing Mind: How Relationships and the Brain Interact to Shape Who We Are.* New York: Guilford Press.

Silverman, D.K. (1998) The tie that binds. *Psychoanalytic Psychology 15*, 187–212.

Slade, A., Cohen, L.J., Sadler, L.S. and Miller, M. (2009) The psychology and psychopathology of pregnancy: Reorganization and transformation. In C.H. Zeanah (ed.) *Handbook of Infant Mental Health*, 3rd edn. New York: Guilford Press.

Smart, C., Strathdee, G., Watson, S., Murgatroyd, C. and McAllister-Williams, R.H. (2015) Early life trauma, depression and the glucocorticoid receptor gene: An epigenetic perspective. *Psychological Medicine 45*, 3393–3410.

Solomon, M.F. and Siegel, D.J. (2003) *Healing Trauma: Attachment, Mind, Body and Brain.* New York: Norton.

Sori, C.F. and Hecker, L.L. (2015) Ethical and legal considerations when counselling children and families. *Australian and New Zealand Journal of Family Therapy 36*, 450–464.

Soundy, C.S. (2009) Young children's imaginative play: Is it valued in Montessori classrooms? *Early Childhood Education Journal 36*, 381–383.

Sovik, R. and Bhavanani, A.B. (2016) History, philosophy and practice of yoga. In S.B.S. Khalsa, L. Cohen, T. McCall and S. Telles (eds) *The Principles and Practice of Yoga in Health Care.* Fountainhall: Handspring Publishing.

Stearns, P. (2015) Children in history. In R.M. Lerner, M.H. Bornstein, T. Leventhal, and R.M. Lerner (eds) *Handbook of Child Psychology and Developmental Science*, 7th edn. New York: Wiley.

Stern, D. (1985) *The Interpersonal World of the Infant: A View from Psychoanalysis and Developmental Psychology.* New York: Basic Books.

Stern, D. (2005) Intersubjectivity. In E.S. Person, A.M. Cooper, and G.O. Gabbard (eds) *Textbook of Psychoanalysis* (pp.77–92). Washington, DC: American Psychiatric Publishing.

Sue, D.W. and Sue, D. (2016) *Counseling the Culturally Diverse: Theory and Practice*, 7th edn. Hoboken, NJ: Wiley.

Sweeney, D.S., Baggerly, J.N. and Ray, D.C. (2014) *Group Play Therapy: A Dynamic Approach.* New York: Routledge.

Taylor, S. and Workman, L. (2018) *The Psychology of Human Social Development: From Infancy to Adolescence.* New York: Routledge.

Terr, L. (1990) *Too Scared to Cry: How Trauma Affects Children and Ultimately Us All.* New York: Basic Books.

Tervalon, M. and Murray-Garcia, J. (1998) Cultural humility versus cultural competency: A critical distinction in defining physician training outcomes in multicultural education. *Healthcare for the Poor and Underserved 9, 2,* 117–125.

Thoenes, C. (2016) *Raphael.* Los Angeles, CA: Taschen.

Toth, S.L. and Gravener, J. (2012) Review: Bridging research and practice: relational interventions for maltreated children. *Child and Adolescent Mental Health 17,* 3, 131–138.

Van der Kolk, B. (2014) *The Body Keeps the Score: Brain, Mind and Body in the Healing of Trauma.* New York: Penguin.

Van der Kolk, B. (2018) Safety and reciprocity: Polyvagal theory as a framework for understanding and treating developmental trauma. In S.W. Porges and D. Dana (eds) *Clinical Applications of the Polyvagal Theory: The Emergence of Polyvagal-Informed Therapies.* New York: Norton.

Van der Kolk, B. and McFarlane, A.C. (1996) The black hole of trauma. In B.A. Van der Kolk, A.C. McFarlane and L. Weisaeth (eds) *Traumatic Stress: The Effects of Overwhelming Experience on Mind, Body and Society.* New York: Guilford Press.

VanFleet, R. and Faa-Thompson, T. (2017) *Animal Assisted Play Therapy.* Sarasota, FL: Professional Resource Press.

Van Rosmalen, L., Van der Veer, R. and Van der Horst, F. (2015) Ainsworth's strange situation procedure: The origin of the instrument. *Journal of the History of Behavioral Sciences 51,* 3, 261–284.

Wang, C.T. and Holton, J. (2007) *Total Estimated Cost of Child Abuse and Neglect in the United States: Economic Impact Study.* Chicago: Prevent Child Abuse America.

Weiner, D.J. (1999) *Beyond Talk Therapy: Using Movement and Expressive Techniques in Clinical Practice.* Washington, DC: American Psychological Association.

Winnicott, D.W. (1953) *Playing and Reality.* London: Tavistock.

Whitaker, R. and Cosgrove, L. (2015) *Psychiatry under the Influence: Institutional Corruption, Social Injury and Prescriptions for Reform.* New York: Palgrave Macmillan.

Woodside, M. (2009) *Thomas Edison: The Man Who Lit Up the World.* New York: Sterling Audible Studios.

Yalom, I.D. (2002) *The Gift of Therapy: An Open Letter to a New Generation of Therapists and Their Patients.* New York: HarperCollins.

Zeanah, CH. (2014) *The Handbook of Infant Mental Health,* 3rd edn. New York: Guilford Press.

Zero to Three (2019) 'Early connections last a lifetime.' Retrieved from https://www.zerotothree.org

Further Reading

Brown, S. (2009) *Play: How It Shapes the Brain, Opens the Imagination and Invigorates the Soul*. New York: Avery.

Dix, J. and McClintic, J. (2016) *Imagination Yoga Teacher Training Manual*. Unpublished manuscript.

Fine, A.H. and Beck, A. (2010) Understanding our kinship with animals: Input for health care professionals interested in the human/animal bond. In A.H. Fine (ed.) *Handbook on Animal Assisted Therapy: Theoretical Foundations and Guidelines for Practice*, 3rd edn. Burlington, MA: Academic Press Elsevier.

Flanagan, L.M. (2016b) The theory of self-psychology. In J. Berzoff, L.M. Flanagan and P. Hertz (eds) *Inside Out and Outside In: Psychodynamic Clinical Theory and Psychopathology in Contemporary Multicultural Contexts*, 4th edn. Lanham, MD: Rowman & Littlefield.

Gil, E. (2006) *Helping Abused and Traumatized Children: Integrating Directive and Nondirective Approaches*. New York: Guilford Press.

Gil, E. (2015) *Play in Family Therapy*, 2nd edn. New York: Guilford Press.

Goodall, J. and Bekoff, M. (2002) *The Ten Trusts: What We Must Do to Care for the Animals We Love*. San Francisco, CA: Harper.

Goodyear-Brown, P. (2010) *Play Therapy with Traumatized Children: A Prescriptive Approach*. Hoboken, NJ: Wiley.

Goodyear-Brown, P., Fath, A. and Myers, L. (2012) Child sexual abuse: The scope of the problem. In P. Goodyear-Brown (ed.) *Handbook of Child Sexual Abuse: Identification, Assessment and Treatment*. Hoboken, NJ: Wiley.

Homeyer, L.E. and Sweeney, D.S. (2011) *Sandtray Therapy: A Practical Manual*, 2nd edn. New York: Routledge.

Khalsa, S.B.S., Telles, S., Cohen, L. and McCall, T. (2016) Introduction to yoga in health care. In S.B.S. Khalsa, L. Cohen, T. McCall and S. Telles (eds) *The Principles and Practice of Yoga in Health Care*. Fountainhall: Handspring Publishing.

Landreth, G.L. (1991) *Play Therapy: The Art of the Relationship*. Muncie, IN: Accelerated Development Publishing.

Malchiodi, C.A. (2008) Creative interventions and childhood trauma. In C.A. Malchiodi (ed.) *Creative Interventions with Traumatized Children*. New York: Guilford Press.

Malchiodi, C.A. (2012) Art therapy and the brain. In C.A. Malchiodi (ed.) *Handbook of Art Therapy*, 2nd edn. New York: Guilford Press.

Presti, D.E. (2016) *Foundational Concepts in Neuroscience: A Brain-Mind Odyssey*. New York: Norton.

Ray, D.C. (2011) *Advanced Play Therapy: Essential Conditions, Knowledge, and Skills for Child Practice*. New York: Routledge.

Ray, D.C. (2016) An overview of child development. In D.C. Ray (ed.) *A Therapist's Guide to Child Development: The Extraordinarily Normal Years*. New York: Routledge.

Satir, V. (1983) *Conjoint Family Therapy*, 3rd edn. Palo Alto, CA: Science and Behavior Books.

Schaefer, C.E. (2011) *Foundations of Play Therapy*, 2nd edn. Hoboken, NJ: Wiley.

Schore, A.N. (2012) *The Science of the Art of Psychotherapy*. New York: Norton.

Siegel, D.J. (2003) An interpersonal neurobiology of psychotherapy: The developing mind and the resolution of trauma. In M.F. Solomon and D.J. Siegel (eds) *Healing Trauma: Attachment, Mind, Body, and Brain*. New York: Norton.

Solomon, M.F. and Siegel, D.J. (2003) *Healing Trauma: Attachment, Mind, Body, and Brain*. New York: Norton.

Terr, L. (1990) *Too Scared to Cry: How Trauma Affects Children and Ultimately Us All*. New York: Basic Books.

Zero to Three (2016) DC: 0–5 Diagnostic classification of mental health and developmental disorders of infancy and early childhood. Washington, DC: Zero to Three.

About the Authors

Michelle Pliske is a licensed clinical social worker (LCSW), the chief executive officer and clinical director for Firefly Counseling Services, P.C. and the director of operations at the Firefly Institute of Research and Education. Michelle is a board recognized supervisor for the Oregon Board of Licensed Clinical Social Workers, Licensed Marriage and Family Therapists and Licensed Professional Counselors. She studied developmental psychology at the University of Washington, Department of Psychology, and at Portland State University, receiving a degree in the School of Social Work. Michelle is a doctoral candidate at the University of Pennsylvania School of Social Work and Social Policy, working towards her Doctor of Clinical Social Work practice with research focused on expressive arts and play therapy to address childhood adverse life experiences. Michelle holds certificates of education in Trauma Informed Services, Adoption and Foster Care, EMDR, and animal assisted human health and is recognized as a Registered Play Therapy Supervisor (RPT-S) through The Association for Play Therapy. She currently works in partnership with Apollo and Mercury, therapy dogs at the institute. Michelle is a certified children's yoga instructor through Imagination Yoga. She is a member of the American Counseling Association (ACA), Association for Play Therapy (APT) and the National Association for Social Workers (NASW). Michelle is a board member for the National Association of Social Workers (NASW) Oregon as vice president.

Lindsay Balboa is a licensed clinical social worker (LCSW) through the Oregon State Board of Licensed Clinical Social Workers. She is also the continuing education director for the Firefly Institute of Research and Education. Lindsay received her bachelor's degree in human development and family sciences with a specialization in early childhood development from the University of Texas at Austin School of Human Ecology. Lindsay received her Master of Science in social work from the University of Texas at Austin Graduate School of Social Work with advanced coursework in child development and play therapy practices. Lindsay works in partnership with Olive and has received training and certification in animal assisted human health. Lindsay has received additional training and post-graduate certification in Adoption and Foster Care and Infant and Toddler Mental Health. Lindsay is certified through Imagination Yoga as a child yoga instructor and she is a member of the Association for Play Therapy.

Subject Index

Sub-headings in *italics* indicate figures and
tables.

acceptance and commitment therapy
(ACT) 73
adverse childhood experiences (ACEs)
15–18
adverse experiences and the nervous
systems 66–8
attachment disruption 51–3
brain development 63–4
brain function 56–8, 62
defining adverse childhood experiences
(ACEs) 47–51
development disruption 53–8
epigenetic considerations 64–6
evidence-based practice 58–61
expressive therapies and movement
61–3
misdiagnosis 58
moment to think activity 71–2
post-traumatic stress disorder (PTSD)
69–70
Ainsworth, Mary 52
animals in therapy 87
animal assisted interventions (AAI) 88
animal assisted neurobiologically
informed play therapy (AANPT)
89–95
animal assisted therapy (AAT) 87–8,
117–19
using animal narratives in the
curriculum 142
Anna 113–21

art 43–5
developmental progression of children's
art 36–9
play therapy and art in clinical practice
45–6
assessment 85
Kelly 108–10
Association for Play Therapy 158
associative play 35
attachment disruption 51–3
attention deficit hyperactivity disorder
(ADHD) 58
autocatalytic model 82–6
Autocatalytic model of practice 86
*Autocatalytic quadripartite assessment
(AQA) of child trauma* 84
therapeutic use of animals 87–95
autonomic nervous system (ANS) 66, 68,
75
Axline, Virginia 43

behavioral problems 62–3
brain function 52–3, 63–4
adverse childhood experiences (ACEs)
56–8, 62
breathing 74–5, 79
burnout 160–1

caregiving 51–2
case studies *see* Anna; Emily; Kelly
central nervous system (CNS) 66, 67
child development 23–5
birth to three years old 25
development disruption 53–8

child development *cont.*
  Erikson's psychosocial theory of
      development 26–7
  Gesell's maturational theory 26
  Greenspan's emotional development
      theory 30–1
  Kohlberg's moral development theory
      29–30
  Piaget's cognitive theory 27–8
  play therapy 32–43
  play therapy and art in clinical practice
      45–6
  prenatal period 25
  six to eleven years old 25
  therapeutic art 43–5
  Vygotsky's cognitive development
      theory 29
children 13–14, 20–2
  adversity and society 15–18
  autocatalytic model 82–6
  children and yoga poses 78–9
  connection 14–15
  holding space for children who suffer
      18–20
children's art 36–9
  consolidating (six to nine years) 37–8
  forming (two to three years) 37
  manipulating (one to two years) 37
  naming (three to four years) 37
  naturalizing (nine to twelve years) 38
  personalizing (twelve to eighteen years)
      38
  representing (four to six years) 37
cognitive development theory 27–9
compassion fatigue 161–3
cooperative play 35–6
countertransference 164–5
cultural humility 23–4

Department of Human Services (DHS) 126
development theory 31–2
  overview of development models 26–32
*Diagnostic and Statistical Manual of Mental
    Disorders (DSM)* 60, 69
directive play therapy 45–6
disclosure 112
divorce 50–1, 53
  work with children experiencing
      divorce 141–2, 144–7, 147–8,
      149–52
dogs 61, 88–95, 142, 144

Edison, Thomas 162
education 157–9
Einstein, Albert 33
Emily 125–33
emotional development theory 30–1
enteric nervous system 67
epigenetics 64–6, 95, 110
Erikson, Erik 26–7
ethical considerations 140, 154–5, 158
  use of animals in therapy 94–5, 159
evidence-based practice 58–61
expressive therapies 18–19, 61
  "Capturing Our Superpowers through
      Creative Capes" 147–8
eye movement desensitization and
    reprocessing (EMDR) 77

family therapy 135–8
  benefits and ethical considerations
      154–5
  family play genograms 99–108
  family yoga interview 138–40
Freud, Anna 40
Freud, Sigmund 39

genetic influences 64–6
Gesell, Arnold 26
Gil, Eliana 13
Greenspan, Stanley 30–1
group work 140
  benefits and ethical considerations
      154–5
  "Calm and Stormy Times" 149–52
  "Capturing Our Superpowers through
      Creative Capes" 147–8
  children experiencing divorce 141–2
  narrative and artful play 152
  "Staying Dry in a Feelings Storm" 152–4
  "The New Pup in Town" 144–7
  using animal narratives in the
      curriculum 142
  using yoga and play 143–4

Harlow, Harry 52
hormones 49, 56–7
Hug-Hellmuth, Hermine 39

Imagination Yoga 143
integration 112–13
intimate partner violence (IPV) 48–9, 53

Kelly 47–51, 97–9
  assessment 108–10
  disclosure 112
  family play genograms 99–108
  integration 112–13
  parent–child interactive therapy (PCIT) 53–5, 60
  treatment planning 110–12
Klein, Melanie 39–40
Kohlberg, Lawrence 29–30
Kohut, Heinz 89

Landreth, Gary 111
Lowenfeld, Margaret 121

maturational theory 26
mind–body connection 14, 21, 157–8
mindfulness 74, 75–7
mindfulness-based stress reduction (MBSR) 76
misdiagnosis 58
Montessori, Maria 33–4
moral development theory 29–30

nervous systems 66–8
  Chart of sympathetic and parasympathetic nervous system 67
neurobiology 18, 20, 22, 46, 62, 85, 110, 158
  neuroception 68
  neurosequential model of therapeutics (NMT) 18, 70
  therapeutic use of animals 87–95, 117–18
non-directive play therapy 45–6

occupational therapy 29, 41, 49–50, 55, 62, 102, 166
onlooker play 36
organizational change 165–6
Osler, Sir William 83

Paper Tigers 19
parallel play 35
parasympathetic nervous system 66, 67, 68, 75, 79, 91–2, 152
parent–child interactive therapy (PCIT) 53–5, 60
Parten, Mildred 35
Patanjali 72

peripheral nervous system (PNS) 66, 67
Piaget, Jean 27–8
Plato 34
play styles 35–6
play therapy 32
  benefits and ethical considerations 154–5
  "Capturing Our Superpowers through Creative Capes" 147–8
  clinical practice 45–6
  definitions of play therapy 43
  developmental progression of children's art 36–9
  developmental progression of play 34–6
  early pioneers in psychotherapy play applications 39–40
  group work 140–2
  importance of play 40–1
  play environments as a grounding principle 32–4
  play in the context of therapy 41–3
  "Staying Dry in a Feelings Storm" 152–4
  using yoga and play 143–4
  yoga and play for therapeutic intervention 81–2
post-traumatic stress disorder (PTSD) 69–70
Psychoanalytic Society 39
psychosocial development theory 26–7

Quebec Suicide Brain Bank 65

Raphael 34
Rogers, Carl 43
Rogers, Fred 165
Rousseau, Jean-Jacques 32, 34, 39

sandtray 121–5
  miniatures 123–4
Satir, Virginia 136–7
scaffolding 29, 30–1
self-care 164–5
social change 165–6
solitary play 35
speech language therapy 55, 109, 166
stress hormones 49, 56–7
sympathetic nervous system 66, 67, 68, 75, 79, 91–2, 152
system stress 163–4

therapeutic art 43–5
therapists 157
    advancement in education and training
        157–9
    burnout 160–1
    compassion fatigue 161–3
    countertransference and absorbing pain
        164–5
    next steps for continued learning 166–7
    remembering who we are 165
    social and organizational change for
        support 165–6
    system stress 163–4
Theraplay® 46, 137
therapy in practice 97–9, 113–21, 125–33
    assessment 108–10
    disclosure 112
    family play genograms 99–108
    integration 112–13
    sandtray 121–5
    treatment planning 110–12
touch 136–7
training 157–9
treatment planning 110–12

United Nations High Commission for
    Human Rights 32
unoccupied play 35

Vygotsky, Lev 29, 35, 43

Wells, H.G. *Floor Games* 121
Winnicott, Donald 13

yoga 72–7
    eight limbs of yoga 77–81
    Imagination Yoga 143
    Limb eight of yoga practice 81
    Limb five of yoga practice 80
    Limb four of yoga practice 79
    Limb three of yoga practice 79
    Limbs one and two of yoga practice 78
    Limbs six and seven of yoga practice
        80–1
yoga therapy 81–2
    benefits and ethical considerations
        154–5
    "Calm and Stormy Times" 149–52
    children and poses 78–9
    family play 136–8
    family yoga interview 138–40
    group work 140–2
    "The New Pup in Town" 144–7
    using yoga and play 143–4

Zero to Three 31
Zone of Proximal Development 29

Author Index

Abramowitz, C.V. 140
Abrams, S. 40
Agur, A.M.R. 57
Aiello, S.E. 91
Almon, J.W. 33
American Art Therapy Association 44
American Psychiatric Association (APA) 58, 60
American Psychological Presidential Task Force 59
Anda, R.F. 50, 56
Andersen, S.L. 56
Anderson, S.M. 53
Applegate, J.S. 63
Arvidson, J. 56
Axline, V.A. 33, 61, 137

Badenoch, B. 51, 52, 57, 63, 67
Baggerly, J.N. 140
Bascandziev, I. 33
Beck, A. 87
Beck, A.M. 87
Beeferman, D. 140
Bekoff, M. 90
Benedict, H.E. 53
Berg, I.K. 46
Bergen, D. 35
Berger, L.M. 58
Berk, L.E. 25
Berzoff, J. 39
Bhavanani, A.B. 73, 77
Biven, L. 56
Bloom, S.L. 19, 164
Blumenfeld, H. 57

Booth, P.B. 46, 137
Bowlby, J. 51, 52, 60
Bratton, S.C. 33
Briere, J. 61
Brown, B. 14, 41
Brown, K.W. 76
Bury, R.G. 35
Butler, K. 88, 92

Carey, S. 33, 61, 141
Carrion, V.G. 56, 57
Cassidy, J. 51
Cha, S. 49
Champagne, F.A. 49
Cloitre, M. 42
Cordon, S.L. 76
Cosgrove, L. 17, 59
Costin, L.B. 16
Courtois, C.A. 69
Cronholm, P.F. 48

Dalley, A.F. 57
Duhl, B. 137
Duhl, F.J. 137
Drewes, A.A. 40

Ener, L. 25

Faa-Thompson, T. 88
Farragher, B. 164
Felitti, V.J. 47, 56
Ferraro, A.J. 50
Figley, C.R. 161
Findling, J.H. 33, 61

Fine, A.H. 87
Fisher, P.A. 57
Flach, C. 49
Flanagan, L.M. 13, 89
Follette, V.M. 77
Ford, J.D. 42, 69
Fraley, R.C. 141
Freud, S. 39
Freyd, J.J. 69
Friedmann, E. 87
Frost, J.L. 35

Galantino, M.L. 141
Galhavy, R. 141
Galovan, A.M. 141
Gapp, K. 65
Gaskill, R.L. 20, 70, 130
Gedo, P.M. 53
Gerson, R. 99
Gesell, A. 26
Gibbons, K. 75
Gil, E. 15, 42–3, 61, 99, 130, 139
Ginsburg, K.R. 32, 41
Glover, V. 49
Goldberg, A. 65
Goodall, J. 90
Goodyear-Brown, P. 127, 152
Gravener, J. 57, 65
Greenspan, S. 31
Grote-Garcia, S., 35

Harder, V.S. 68
Harker, A. 56, 57, 65, 68
Havener, L. 87
Hayes, S.C. 73
Hecker, L.L. 158
Heffernan, M.E. 141
Hembree-Kigin, T.L. 53, 54
Henderson, D. 33
Henson, R.K. 33
Herman, J.L. 157
Hesse, E. 52
Holton, J. 58
Homeyer, L.E. 122
Hughes, V. 65
Hunt, T.K.A. 58

Irwin, E C. 138
Islam, S.A. 64

Jernberg, A.M. 46, 137
John, M. 83
Johnson, J.L. 15, 39, 40

Kabat-Zinn, J. 76
Kantor, D. 137
Karr-Morse, R. 42
Katcher, A.H. 87
Keshavan, M.S. 57
Kestly, T. 125
Khalsa, S.B.S. 73
Klaff, D. 122
Klein, B.G. 91
Klein, M. 40
KPJR Films Production 19
Kobor, M.S. 64
Kottman, T. 46
Kruger, K.A. 87–8

Labonté, B. 65
Landreth, G.L. 32, 31, 61
Lebo, D. 32, 39, 40
Lemmens, J.S. 16
Levine, P.A. 42, 67
Lillard, A.S. 33
Louv, R. 41
Lussier, A.A. 64

MacNeil, G.A. 18
Main, M. 52
Malchiodi, C.A. 19, 20, 36, 38, 41, 44, 61,
    69, 142
Malloy, E.S. 138
Masho, S.W. 49
Maslach, C. 160
McFarlane, A.C. 42
McGoldrick, M. 99, 136
McNeil, C.B. 53, 54
Meadows, S. 23
Melson, G.F. 87, 89
Mercer, J. 53
Midgley, N. 40
Monk, C. 49
Montessori, M. 34, 43
Moore, D.S. 64
Moore, K.L. 57, 64, 66, 91
Munns, E. 137
Murray-Garcia, J. 24

Newell, J.M. 18
Nolte, J. 63, 64
Nugent, N.R. 65

Oaklander, V. 46
O'Brien, J. 41
O'Connor, K. 46
Orvaschel, H. 140

Panksepp, J. 56
Patterson, J. 136
Pears, K. 57
Peña, C.J. 49
Perry, B.D. 18, 20, 56, 64, 70, 130, 141
Peter, J. 16
Petry, S. 99
Pham, P. N. 15
Polusny, M.A. 76
Porges, S.W. 61, 62, 67–8
Presti, D.E. 63, 66, 67
Purves, D. 63

Quinn, L. 141

Ramo-Fernandez, L. 64
Ray, D.C. 26, 27, 29, 30, 31, 41, 43, 140
Reifel, S.C. 35
Reiss, A.L. 56
Rogers, C. 153
Rousseau, J.J. 32
Rubin, J.A. 36–7

Sandman, C.A. 65
Sapolsky, R.M. 49, 66
Schaefer, C.E. 40, 46
Schore, A.N. 90
Schore, J.R. 90
Schramm, D.G. 141
Schubach De Domenico, G. 122, 123
Schulten, K. 165
Scott, C. 61
Serpell, J.A. 87–8
Shaffer, D.R. 27, 28
Shapiro, F. 77
Shapiro, J.R. 63
Shapiro, S.L. 76
Shelan, W. 41, 61
Shuffelton, A.B. 32
Siegel, D.J. 42, 51, 53, 56, 63, 67, 90, 125

Silverman, D.K. 53
Slack, K.S. 58
Slade, A. 25
Smart, C. 64
Smith, J. 41
Solomon, M.F. 56
Son, H. 87
Sori, C.F. 158
Soundy, C.S. 34
Sovik, R. 73, 77
Stearns, P. 23
Steiner, T. 46
Stern, D. 90
Stewart, A.L. 41, 61
Stover, E. 15
Strosahl, K.D. 73
Sue, D. 48
Sue, D.W. 48
Sweeney, D.S. 122, 140

Taylor, S. 24, 25
Teicher, M.H. 56
Terr, L. 42, 43
Tervalon, M. 24
Thoenes, C. 34
Thompson, C.L. 33
Toth, S.L. 57, 65
Tsai, C.C. 87

Uddin, M. 65

Valkenburg, P.M. 16
Van der Horst, F. 52
Van der Kolk, B. 32, 42, 56, 60, 61, 62, 66, 75
Van der Veer, R. 52
VanFleet, R. 88
Van Rosmalen, L. 52
Vijay, A. 77
Vinck, P. 15

Wang, C.T. 58
Weems, C.F. 56
Weiner, D.J. 18
Wiley, M.S. 42
Winnicott, D.W. 131
Whitaker, R. 17, 59
Wilson, K.G. 73
Wong, S.S. 57

Woodside, M. 162
Workman, L. 24, 25
Wortham, S.C. 35

Yalom, I.D. 41

Zaitchik, D. 33
Zeanah, CH. 56, 57
Zero to Three 31